Little people a pondering?

Mite World

www.miteworld.com

Health & Environment

Read Mite World & Chuckle your way down the Path to Wellness

Packed with Holistic Expert references.

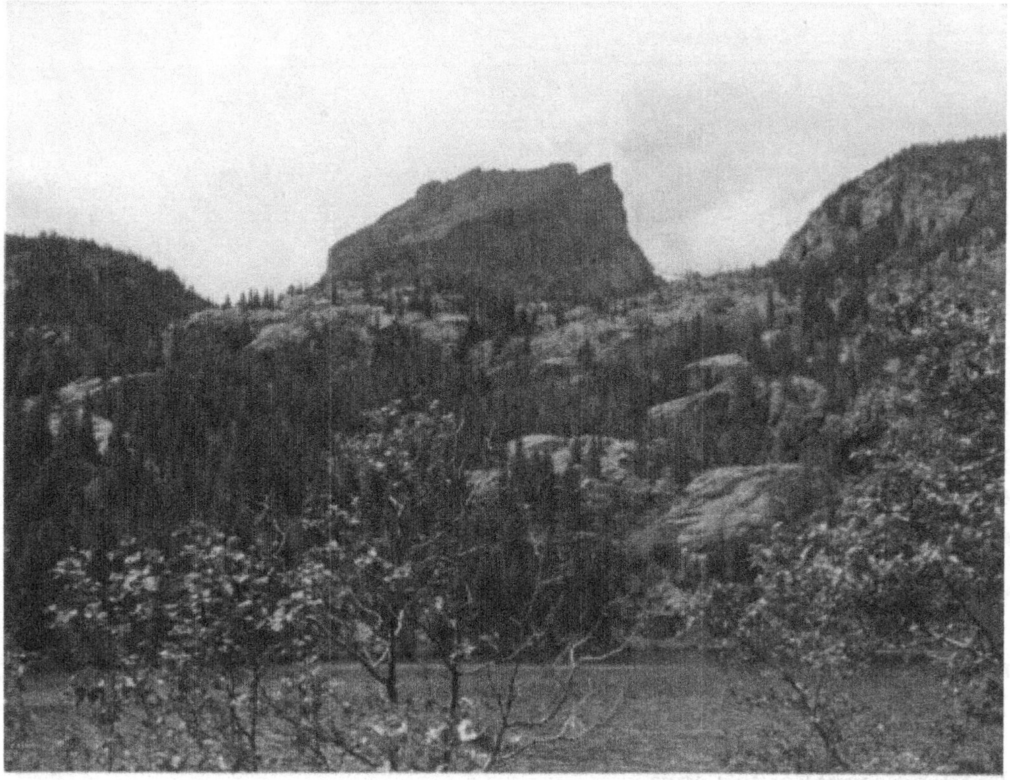

bu Adam J Reissner

ISBN 978-0-7414-1239-3

Published by:

INFINITY PUBLISHING

1094 New DeHaven Street, Suite 100
West Conshohocken, PA 19428-2713
Toll-free (877) BUY BOOK
Local Phone (610) 941-9999
Fax (610) 941-9959
Info@buybooksontheweb.com
www.buybooksontheweb.com

Printed in the United States of America

Published January-2012

Acknowledgments

Special thanks to my loving wife Bonnie, for her help, encouragement, photographic talent and patience for tolerating me hogging the computer to write this book. Many thanks to Mr. Robert Morris for his inspiration by example and steering me to Infinity Publishing, Inc. I wish to express my gratitude to Mr. Dutch Schulz for his photos on the twin towers.

Preface

I'm a medical layman. I believe in pluralistic health care that uses *both* conventional and holistic medicine to achieve and maintain wellness without going bankrupt, as long as decisions made are informed ones. The problem is that an adversary relationship exists between these two groups, creating much confusion; thus making it difficult for us, the little people, who are in the middle. Entrenched in the governmental health departments and insurance companies, condescending conventional practitioners seek to prevent or hinder the holistic people from offering options in health care. The conventional medicine people believe that only they know what is right for all. Why not use the best of both worlds? Therefore, as patients, we reap the benefit. This means being responsible for our own wellness. It requires us to be informed, which includes questioning our health care provider attentively.

Mite World is the sharing of my investigations derived from holistic experts. It is written in an amusing format with minimum technical jargon to invoke the reader's curiosity. This is accomplished by phrasing sarcastic questions with factual responses while interjecting levity along with photos to accentuate the topic. I use abbreviated dialogue between personalities presented in comic-book fashion shown as dots, to illustrate mites, or the little people, who individually are *not* the world's movers and shakers. Emphasis is on health and the environment.

<u>The Cast of characters:</u>

- Albert, the obnoxious, brainy, know-it-all.
- Gracie, Albert's clever, inquisitive and intuitive wife.
- Uncle Billy, Albert's lovable, blasé and obtuse older uncle-in-law.
- Walter, Albert's bright, but sarcastic older brother.

The implied philosophy expressed in this book is that everything in life has a price, though at times the amount and due date are unknown, especially when it comes to health and environmental issues.

Each narrative is a stand-alone vignette best read collectively with the other the narratives. The book is to be read with a facetious attitude while encouraging the reader to become more informed and inquisitive about his wellness, or at least to start contemplating options.

The technical information is derived from many different sources, with the primary sources listed in a bibliography for reference and acknowledgments.

Cast of Characters

These characters are fictitious, and any resemblance to real persons, present or past, is coincidental.

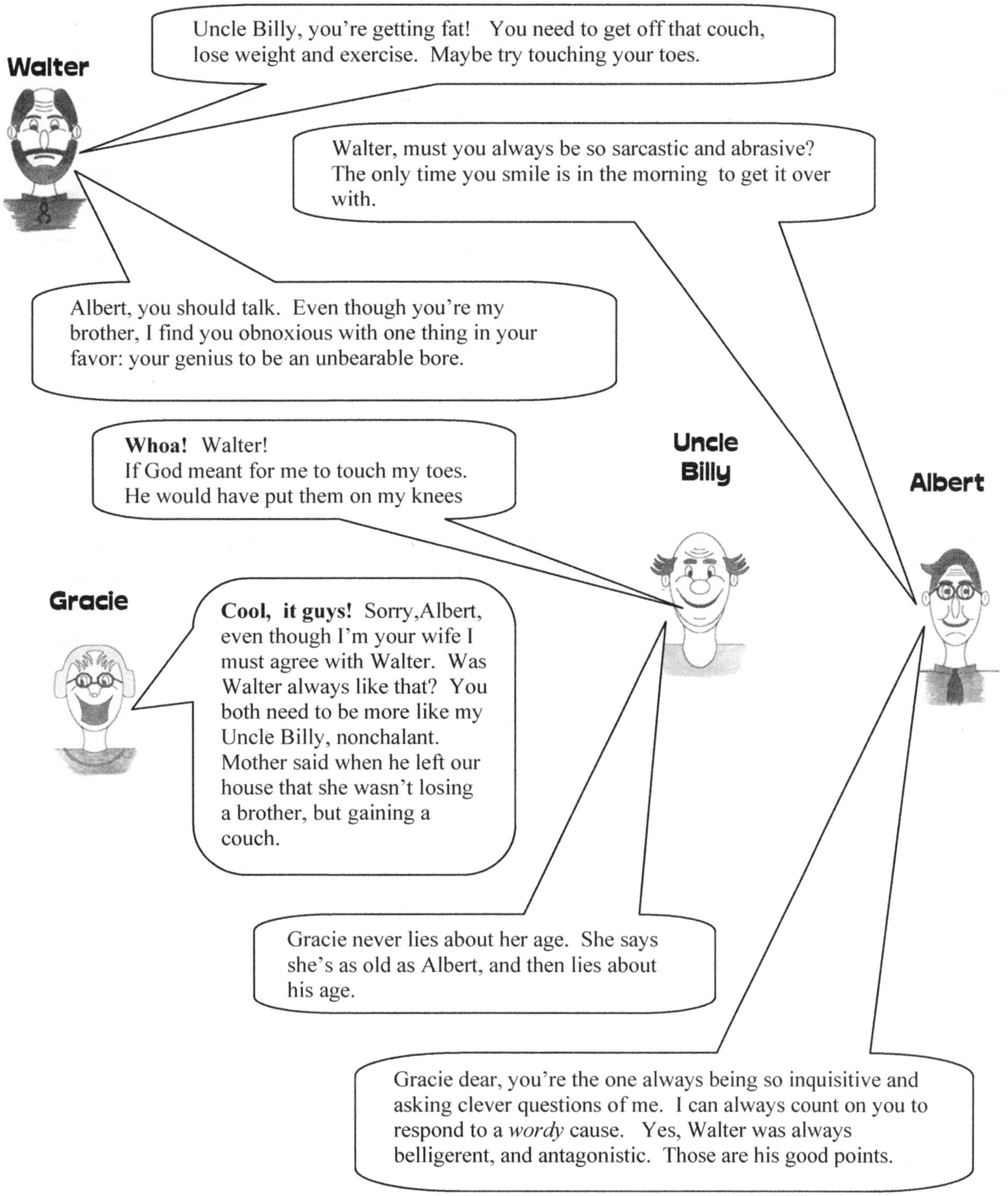

Health Disclaimer

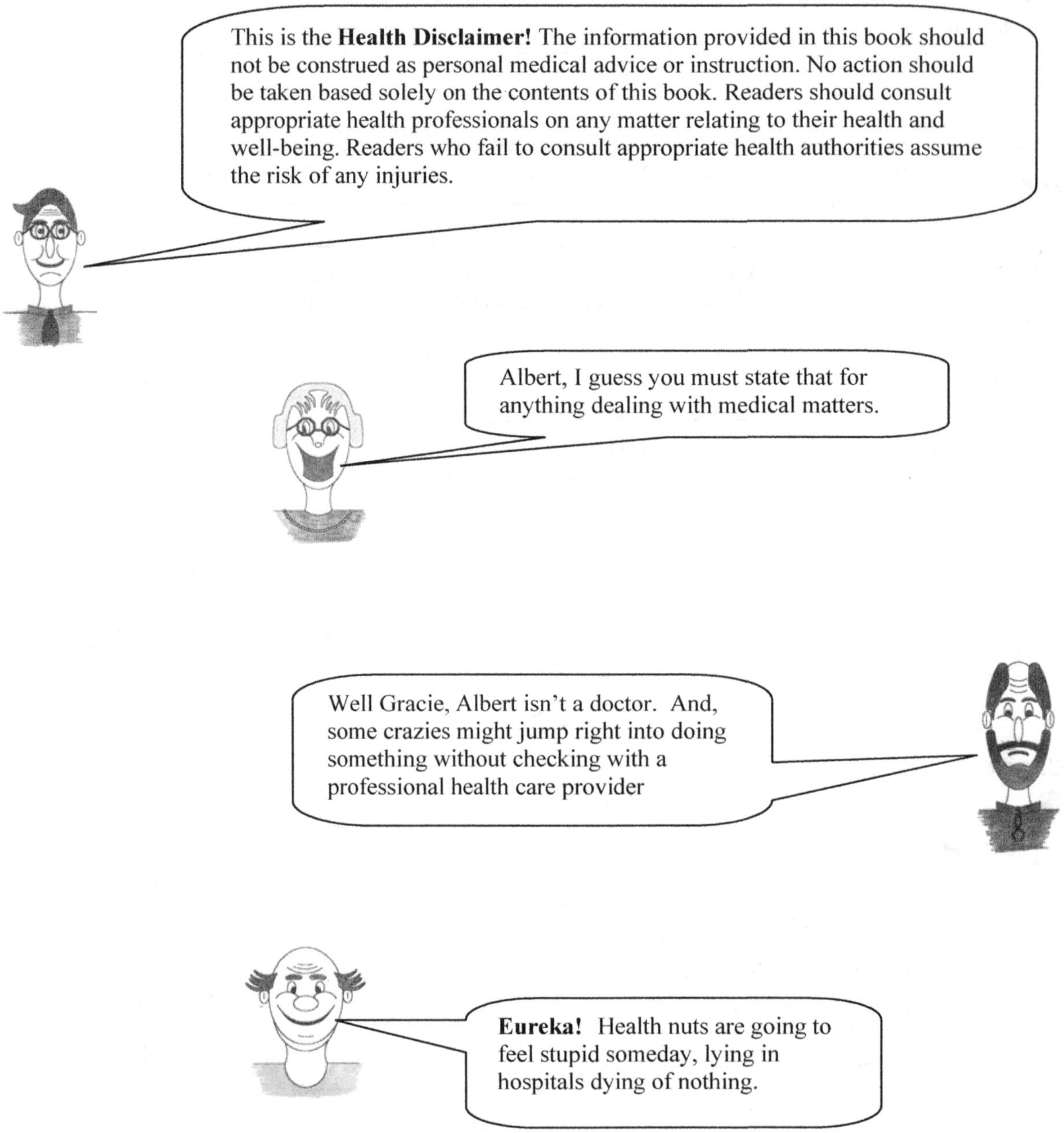

Table of Contents

Health - General

With Medical cost escalating through the roof and prescription drugs emerging more powerful than ever with associated insidious side effects, the need to seek options becomes imperative. Not to supplant conventional wisdom, but to complement it for one's own wellness & being. Self-reliance is the key word to your health. Just a pondering?

Protocol - Pay me now or pay me later.

Practice having a good diet and using natural supplements, or end up with powerful synthetic drugs and surgery.

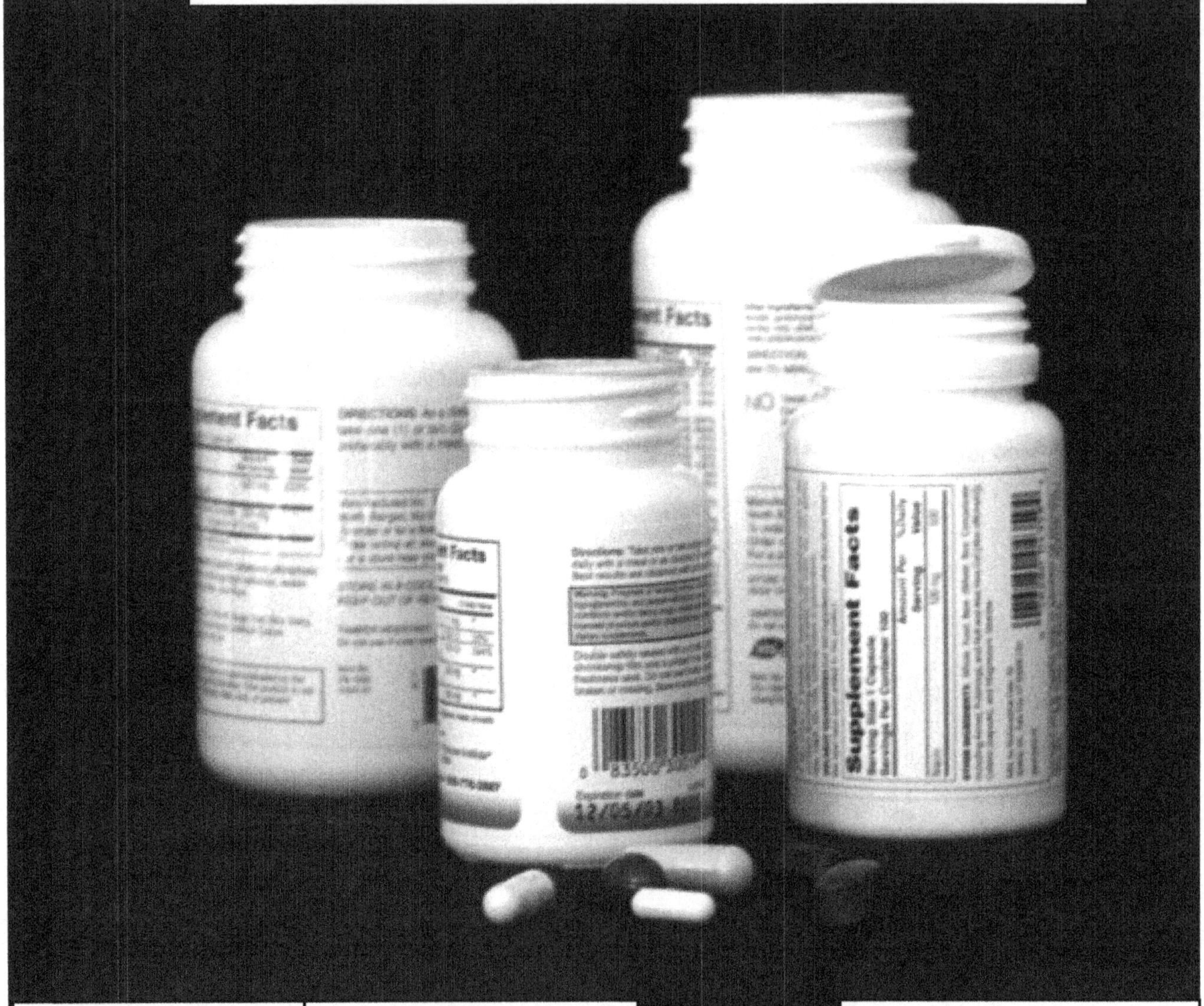

Goodies & Tidbets:

A, B's,C, D, E, coQ10, Garlic, Selenium, Zinc, Calcium, Magnesium, Grape Seed Extract

Site-Search: www.

alternativemedicine.com

Book Bowse:

Alternative Medicine the Definitive Guide, by Goldberg, Burton MD.

Conventional vs. Holistic medicine

Must Health methods collide? NO!

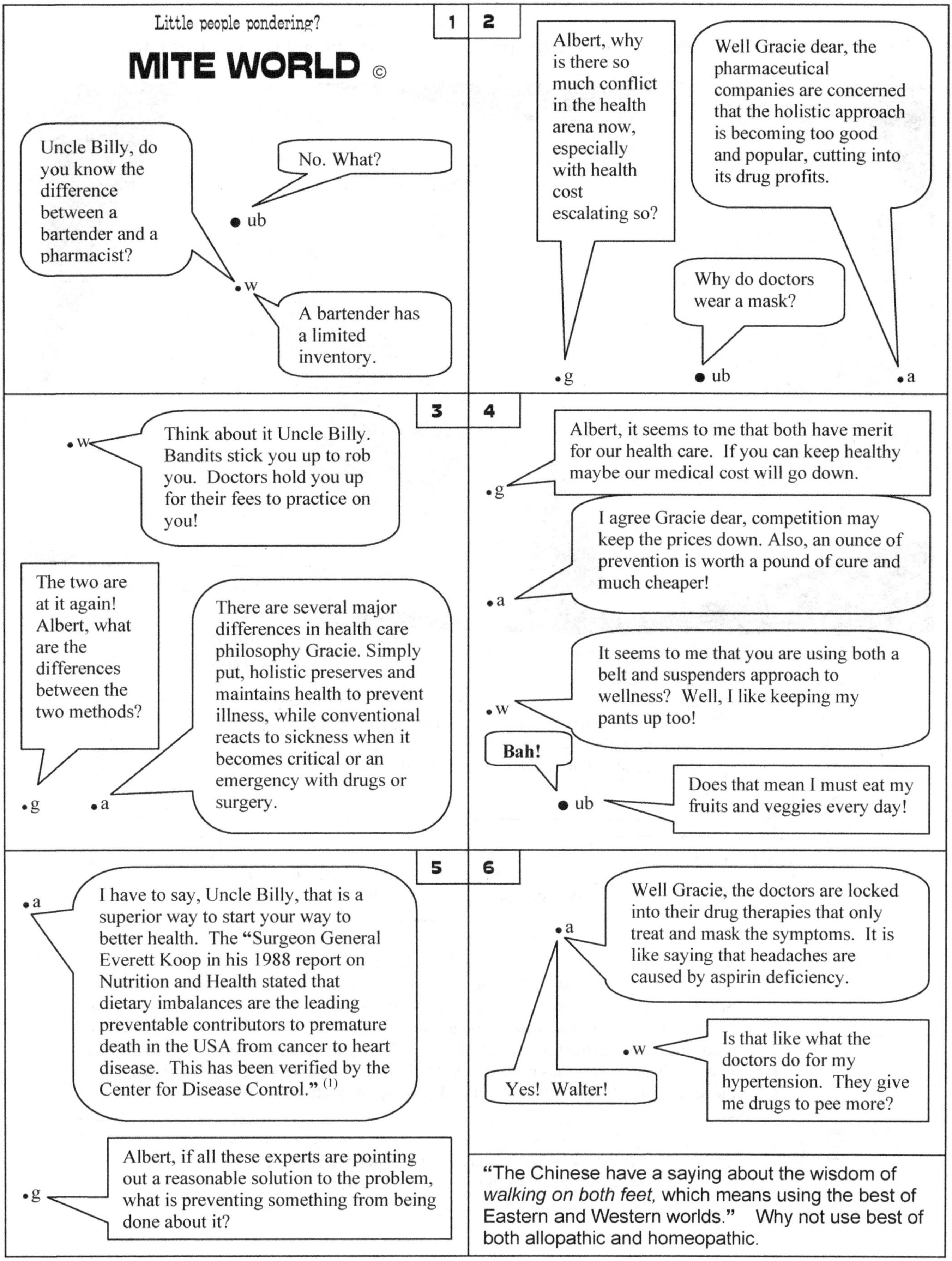

What direction forward or backward - only time will tell.

Shuffling the charts together will merge the past with the present and can obfuscate the future??

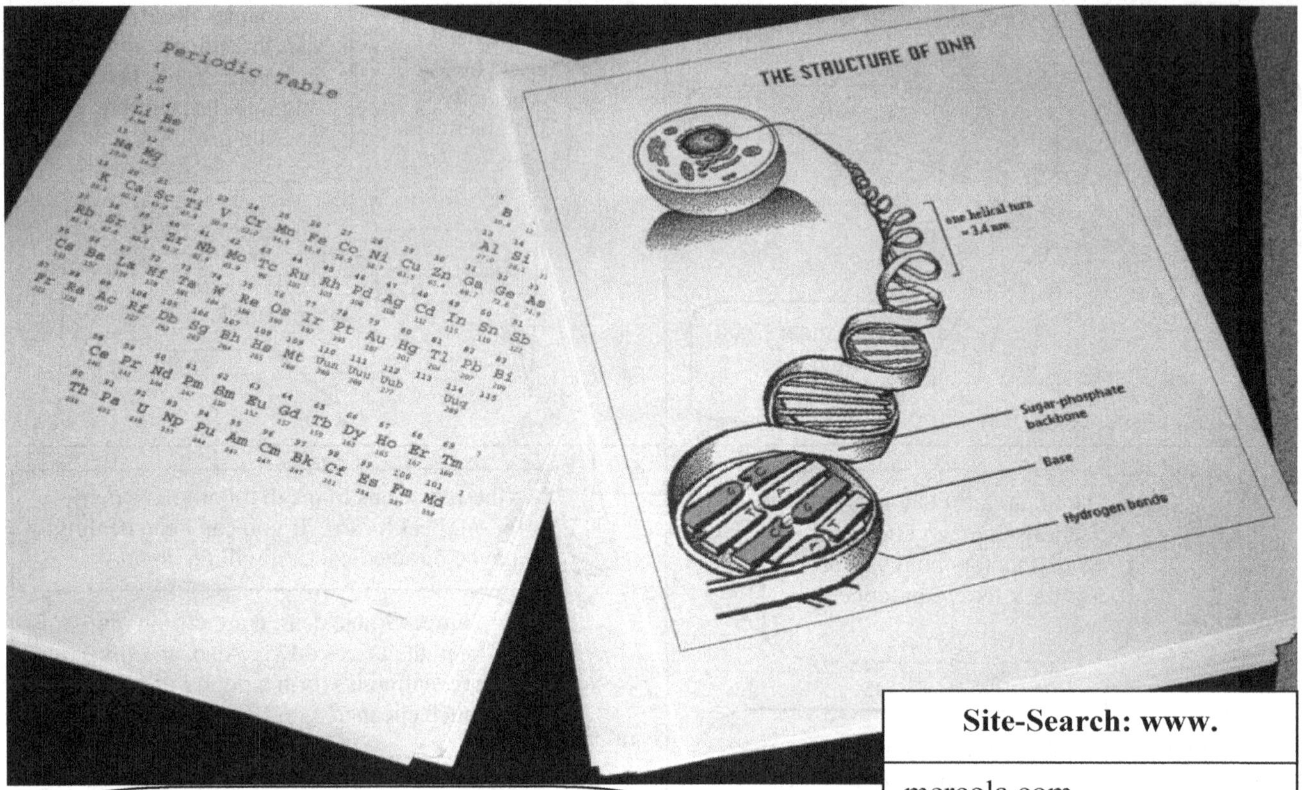

Site-Search: www.

mercola.com
thimersoal-news.com

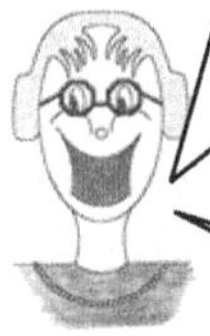

I've been hearing that Autism is on the rise.

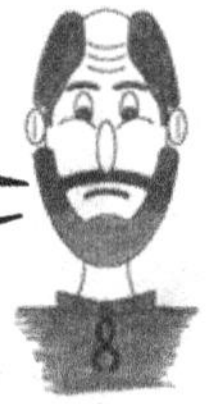

Yeah! There have been several class actions against pharmaceutical companies that produce the drugs for several popular children vaccines that are believed to cause adverse effects such as Autism.

Oh, how horrible!

Vaccines contain Thimerosal, a mercury compound, which is cheap.

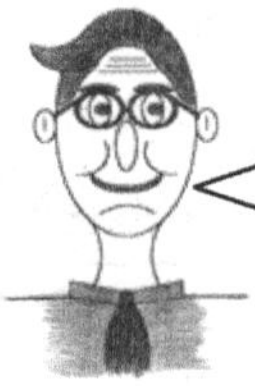

It is Gracie. The researchers believe that Thimerosal, a vaccine preservative and antibacterial compound, is the cause. These vaccines are routinely used for children. Studies have linked Thimerosal to mercury poisoning in infants often causing Autism. Initially they believed that the amounts were so small as to have no adverse effect, but didn't take into account the accumulative influence it could have on small bodies. Keep in mind that **"**all vaccines marketed in the U.S are based on a benefit-to-risk analysis of the safety and efficacy data submitted by the sponsors to the FDA**"** [(2)]

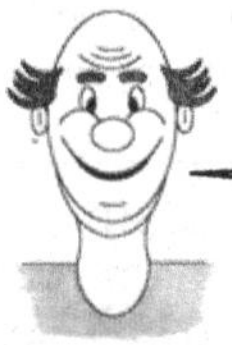

I guess the pharmaceuticals and FDA need to be super cautious. Never make the same mistake once.

Charts - Periodic & Genome

Maps of obliteration or creation?

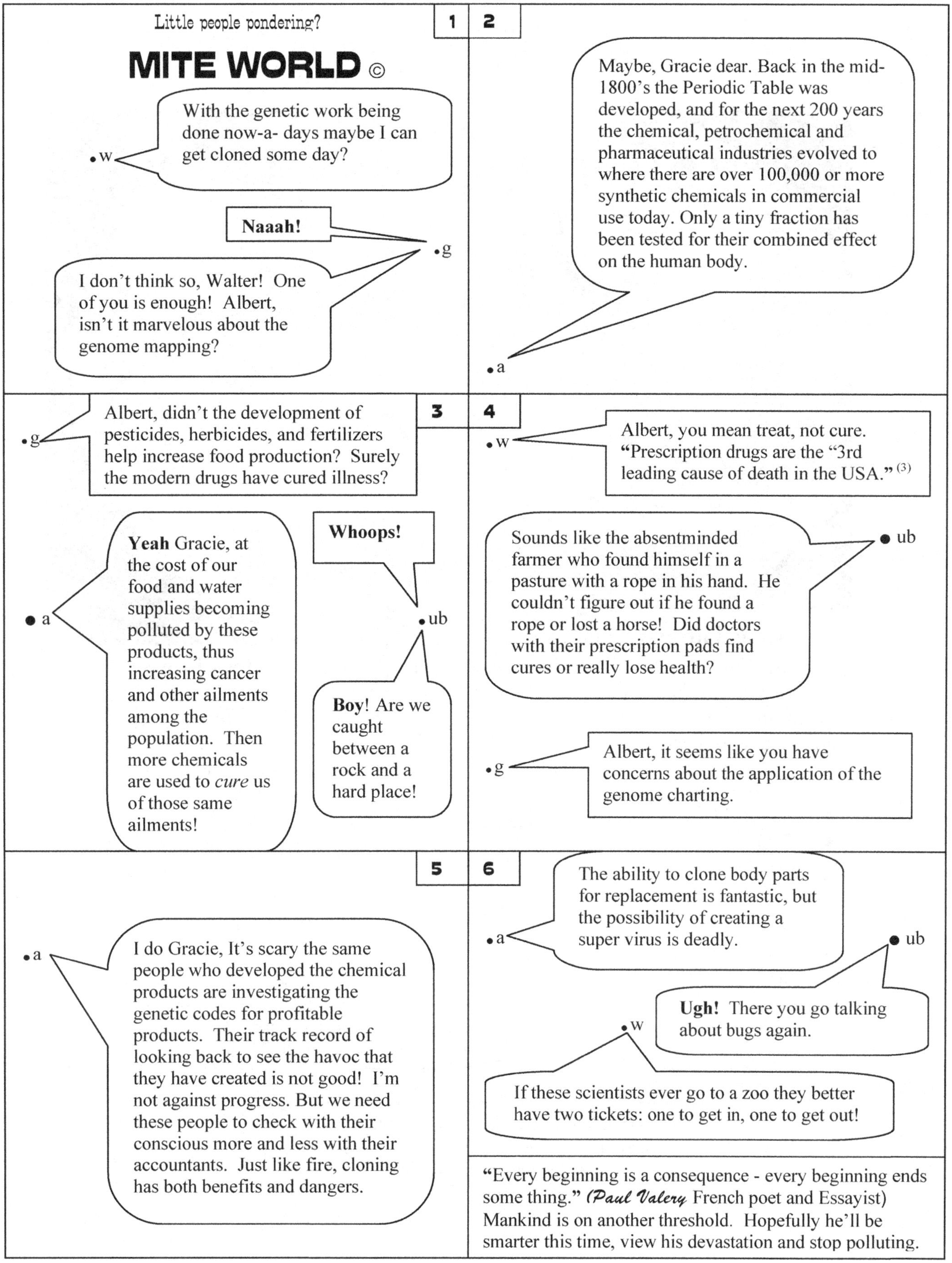

I love eggs- *Clucked full of good stuff.*

Mother Nature's vitamin pill.

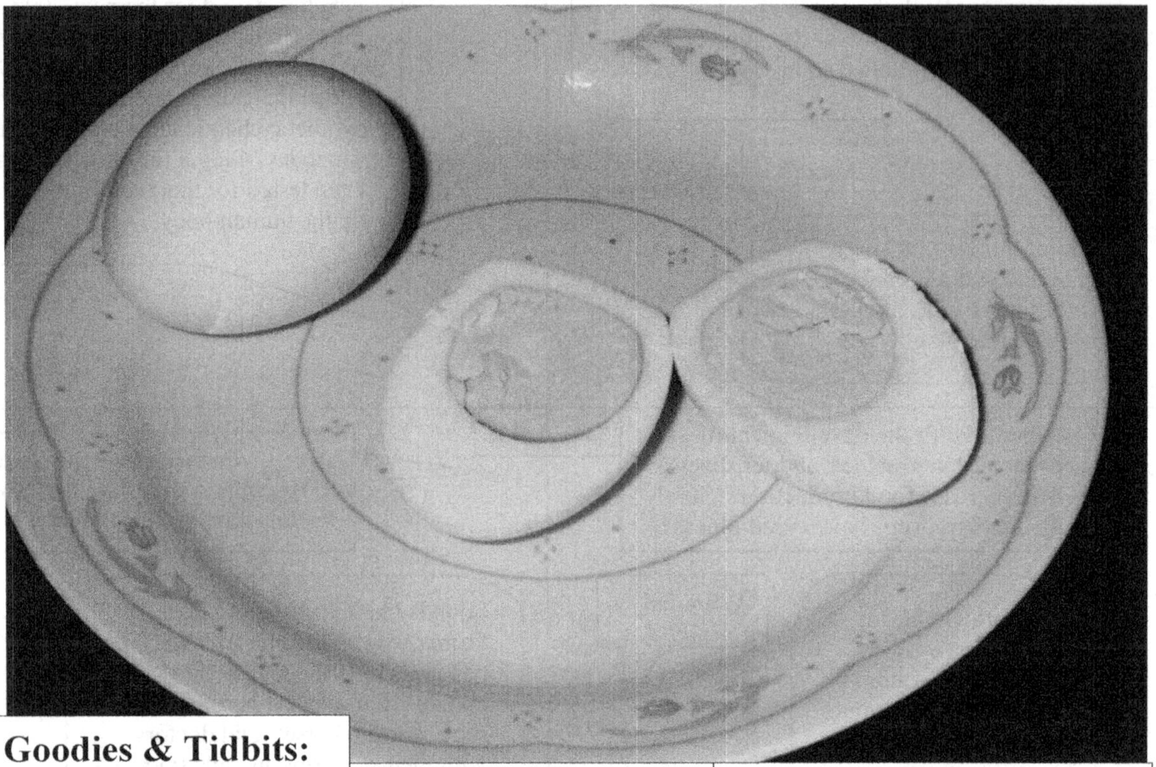

Goodies & Tidbits: *Key Words*	Site-Search: www.	Book Browse
For quantities see bibliography references	drwhitaker.com hsibaltimore.com wholehealthmd.com	*New breakthroughs Against heart disease and stroke;* by Health Sciences Inst. Editorial Panel *Healthy alternatives to the 100 most commonly prescribed drugs;* By Whitaker, Julian MD.

- Vitamin B6
- Vitamin B12
- CoQ10
- Folic acid
- Niacin
- Water
- E-Tocotrienols
- Omega3 Oil
- Lecithin
- Garlic

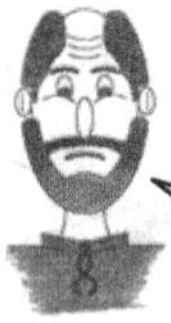

It has been revealed that "drug companies spend nearly twice as much on marketing, advertising and administration as on R&D." (4)

"The FDA has just been alerted of a problem more serious. Statin drugs deplete the body of its CoQ10, which leads to reduction in heart flexibility. This causes more stress on the heart." (4)

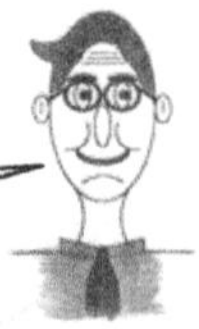

Is Cholesterol the Problem?

homocysteine the real culprit

1

Little people pondering?

MITE WORLD©

w: The doctor said my cholesterol is high and put me on a Statin drug.

g: Sorry Walter, I read that these drugs had "significant side effects, which can cause liver damage, muscle cramps, nausea, constipation, as well as hair loss".(5)

2

w: **Oh no!** The doctor explained most of that to me, stressing that it will help prevent heart disease and stroke. He missed hair loss.

a: Hair loss is a minor side effect, Walter, More serious is that you also have hypertension. A "study has shown that people with hypertension and taking Statin drugs after 6 months experience a decline in their cognitive abilities, attention span and dexterity." (4)

w: **Sigh!** I certainly don't need that to happen. Are there some options I can try to help control my cholesterol?

3

a: Yes there are several complementary nutrients you can use with your prescription, check with your doctor. Start taking "vitamins B6, B12 and folic acid to help reduce the homocysteine in your system." (5)

ub: Is that some kind of disease you get from a gay German?

a: Very funny, Uncle Billy. **No!** Cholesterol needs to be in your blood for proper cell health. The problem occurs when cholesterol builds up on your arteries. This "occurs when there is too much homocysteine, an amino acid, which damages the artery walls allowing for the plaque to collect." (4)

4

a: Eating foods with the B vitamins I mentioned or as supplements can help to keep elevated homocysteine in check and prevent arteriosclerosis.

g: Maybe with time your cholesterol will come down and you can get off the drugs?

w: I sure hope so, but reaching the doctor may be a problem, especially when he said that I could reach his answering machine anytime. Next he gave me his pager in case I can't get the answering machine.

5

a: More important is the need to take the "antioxidant vitamin E in the tocotrienols form, since it is 60% more effective than its' cousin alpha-tocopherol. This E has been found to reduce platelet, clumping and lower cholesterol. It also is a natural blood thinner as well." (4) Another good nutrient is CoQ10.

w: **Gosh**! Albert, you scare the pants off me with all the talk about side affects! Sure hope the vitamin E helps.

6

a: Walter, take heart, no pun intended. "In a double blind human trial, supplementation with a high-potency tocotrienol resulted in significant reductions in cholesterol and LDL levels." (4)

ub: **Yeah**, Walter, you'll be around for a long time just to irritate me.

w: Not only do I want to live long, but also it would be nice to have a decent quality of life. Bugging you, Uncle Billy helps.

All mankind is divided into three classes: Those that are immovable, those that are movable, and those that move.

Arabian Proverb

Exchanging one problem for another

That's a stiff drink! I think?

Don't fool around with Mother Nature casually. Unexpected repercussions result.
X - off the use of fluoride.

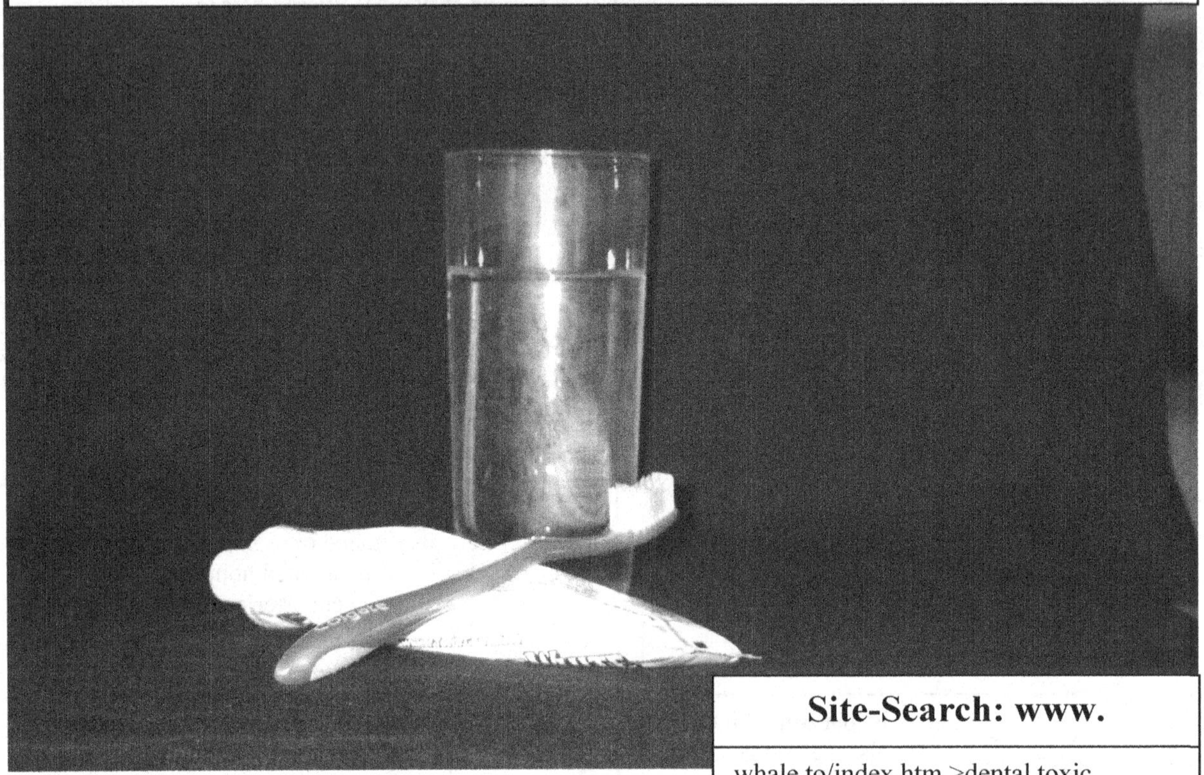

Site-Search: www.

whale.to/index.htm >dental toxic >fluoride

garynull.com >world issues>fluoride

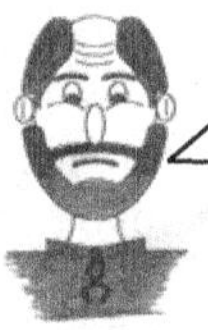

Hey! Albert, I just learned that Canada's leading fluoride authority, Dr. Limeback, who until recently was that country's primary promoter of the controversial additive fluoride, announced a dramatic change of heart. "Children under three should never use fluoridated toothpaste, or drink fluoridated water." [7]

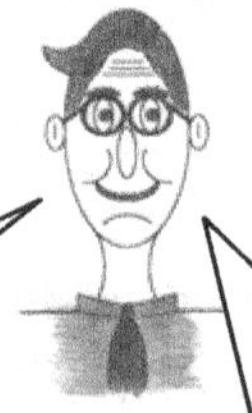

Yeah! Walter, he came to the "realization that they have been dumping contaminated fluoride into water reservoirs for half a century. The vast majority of all fluoride additives come from Tampa Bay smokestack scrubbers. The additives are a toxic byproduct of the super-phosphate fertilizer industry." [7]

Good thinking Gracie! Yes, "deadly elements of lead, arsenic and radium, all of them carcinogenic." [7] It is important that we use good filtration on our water, since water is also a must for hydration of our bodies. We all need to lobby for the elimination of fluoride from our water supply.

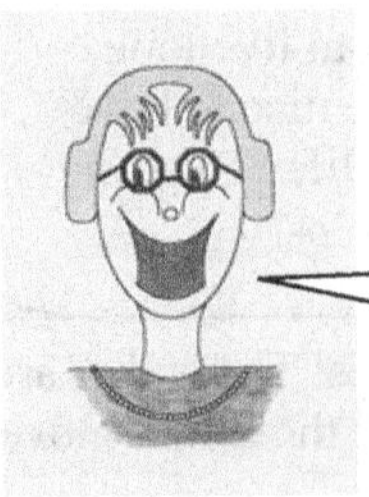

Oh my heavens! That's a waste product. It must mean that other toxins are also included.

Alzheimer's link to fluoridation.

Drinking water prevents cavities if my memory serves me right!

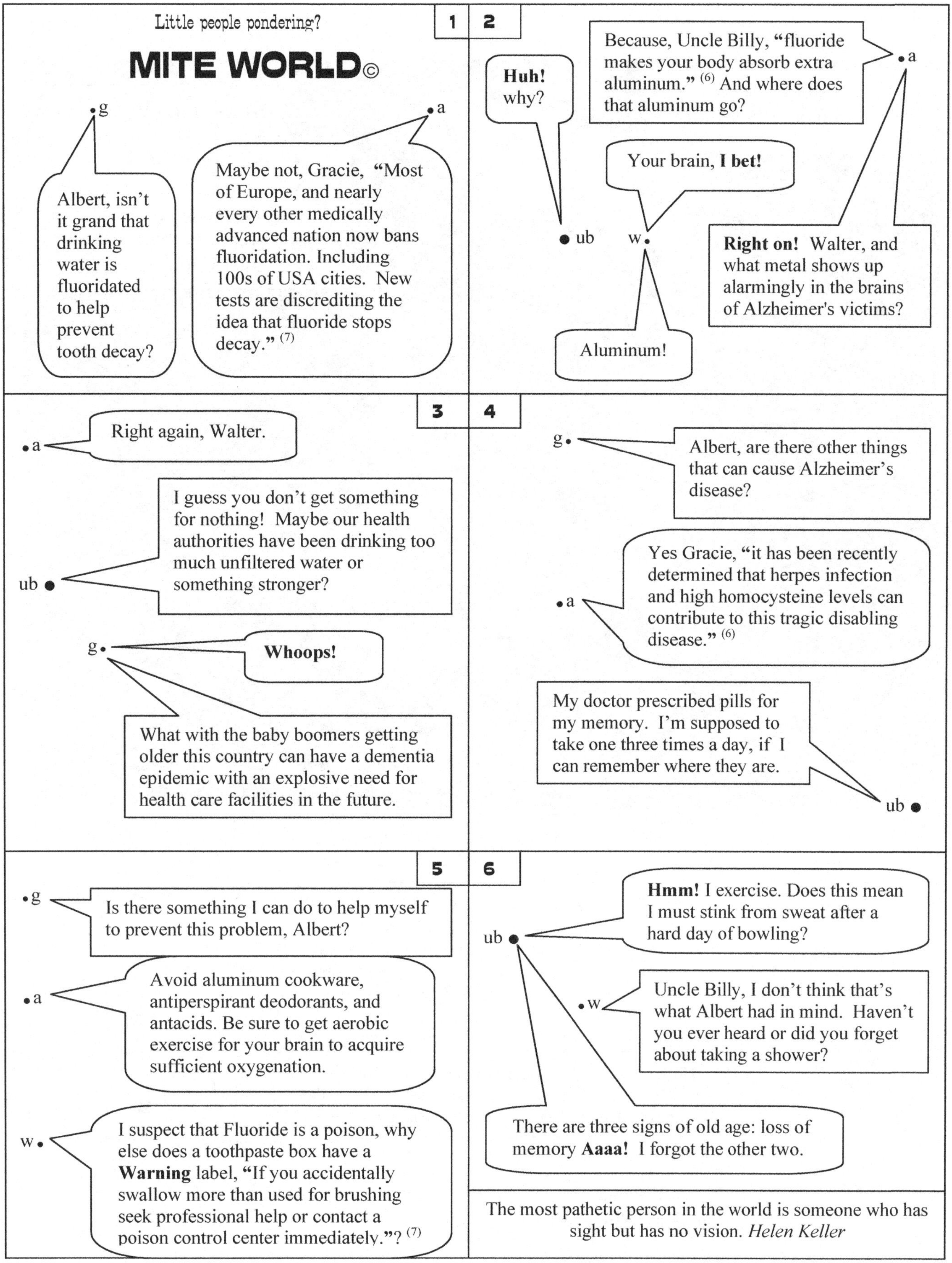

Benefit of smoking???

Converting your lungs to a dirty ashtray

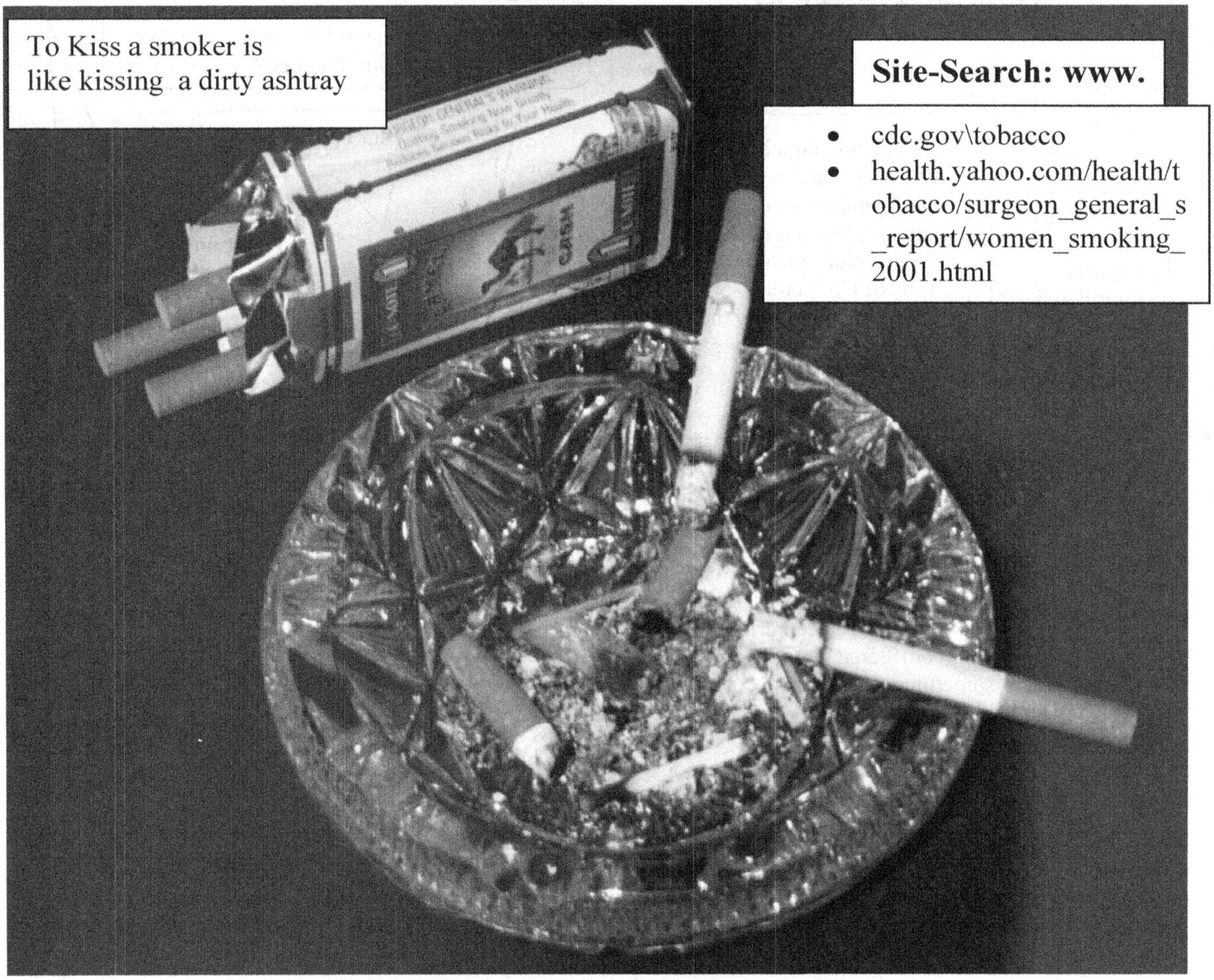

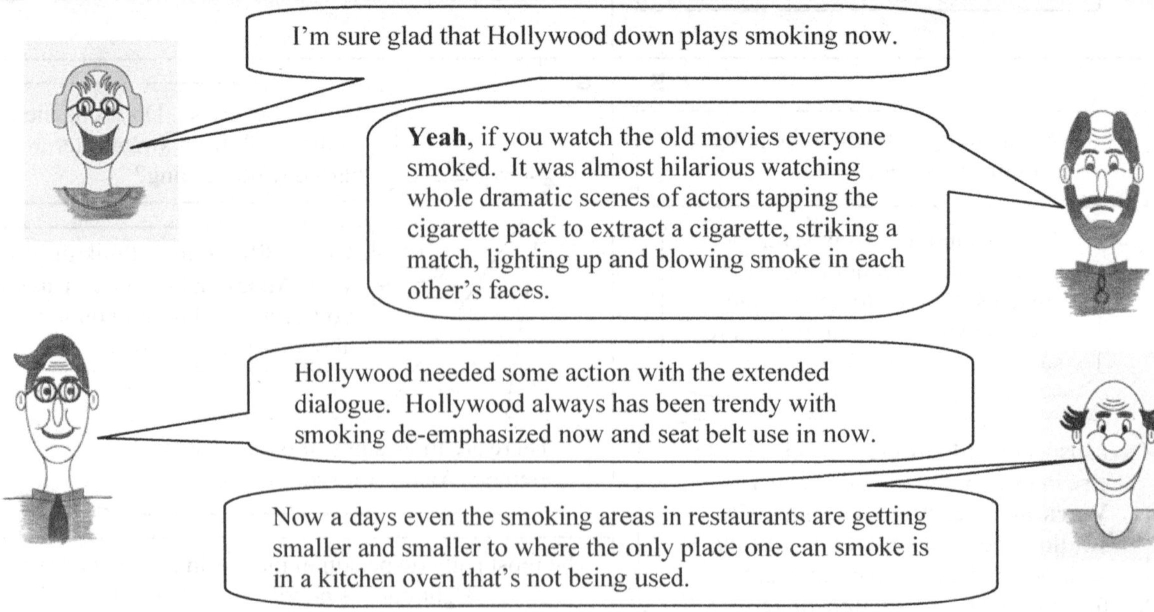

Cigarette Butts

Slobs proliferate!

1

Little people pondering?

MITE WORLD©

w: Uncle Billy, aren't cigarettes called coffin nails?

ub: **Yea,** Walter, and cancer sticks too! Since I've stopped smoking I feel better, I smell better and it's safer to drink from old beer cans around the house.

2

g: Albert, on the roadside where I walk 2miles a day I see cigarette butts all over. Being curious one day I counted the butts on my amble, and to my surprise I counted 75/mile. This litter represents inconsiderate people, as well as a sign of a lot of people tempting ill health.

a: I agree on both counts Gracie, "Tobacco use causes about one of every five deaths in the United States and is the single most preventable cause of death and disease in our nation. This amounts to 430,000 deaths/year." (8)

3

w: I believe people who don't care about their own body cleanliness certainly are not going to worry about littering the countryside.

g: Albert, people caught littering by flipping butts in public should be penalized by having to pick up butts at their own expense. People are now a days more militant against smokers. The warning on the pack should read "Smoking may be injurious to your health. The person next to you may hit you with a stick."

4

a: Right on Gracie dear! Uncle Billy, I'm glad you quit smoking. Too bad we can't stop teens from starting. Of the "3 million young people under age 18 that smoke half a billion cigarettes each year, 1 million of them will die a premature, preventable death because of a decision made as a youngster." (8) Most start smoking because of peer pressure.

ub: **My gosh!**

I quit in my late teens. People were getting rude to smokers. You'd think they'd try to be nicer to those who were dying.

5

g: Albert, tobacco company officers that lied and concealed facts from the public about smoking having no effect on one's health should spend one year in a smoke filled room for their arrogance and sin of poisoning people.

a: Gracie, that will never happen. Too bad! I'm sorry to say that "Prez Bush has just cut the federal funding for the Justice Department's court action against Big Tobacco's 50-year conspiracy." (8)

6

a: These companies deceive us about cigarette addiction and aggressive targeting of kids. "The budget changed from $32 million to $1.8 million." (8)

w: I'm sure glad you have stopped smoking Uncle Billy. Good health is the slowest possible rate one can die, but smoking accelerates that rate.

"Do I get a gold star for my first 100 days?" Bush asked of some college students. Who then ambushed him by standing in front of the White House with placards spelling out, "Pollution Starts Here." With Bush in the white house, Big business will win over the environment every time.

I can't wait- please hurry!

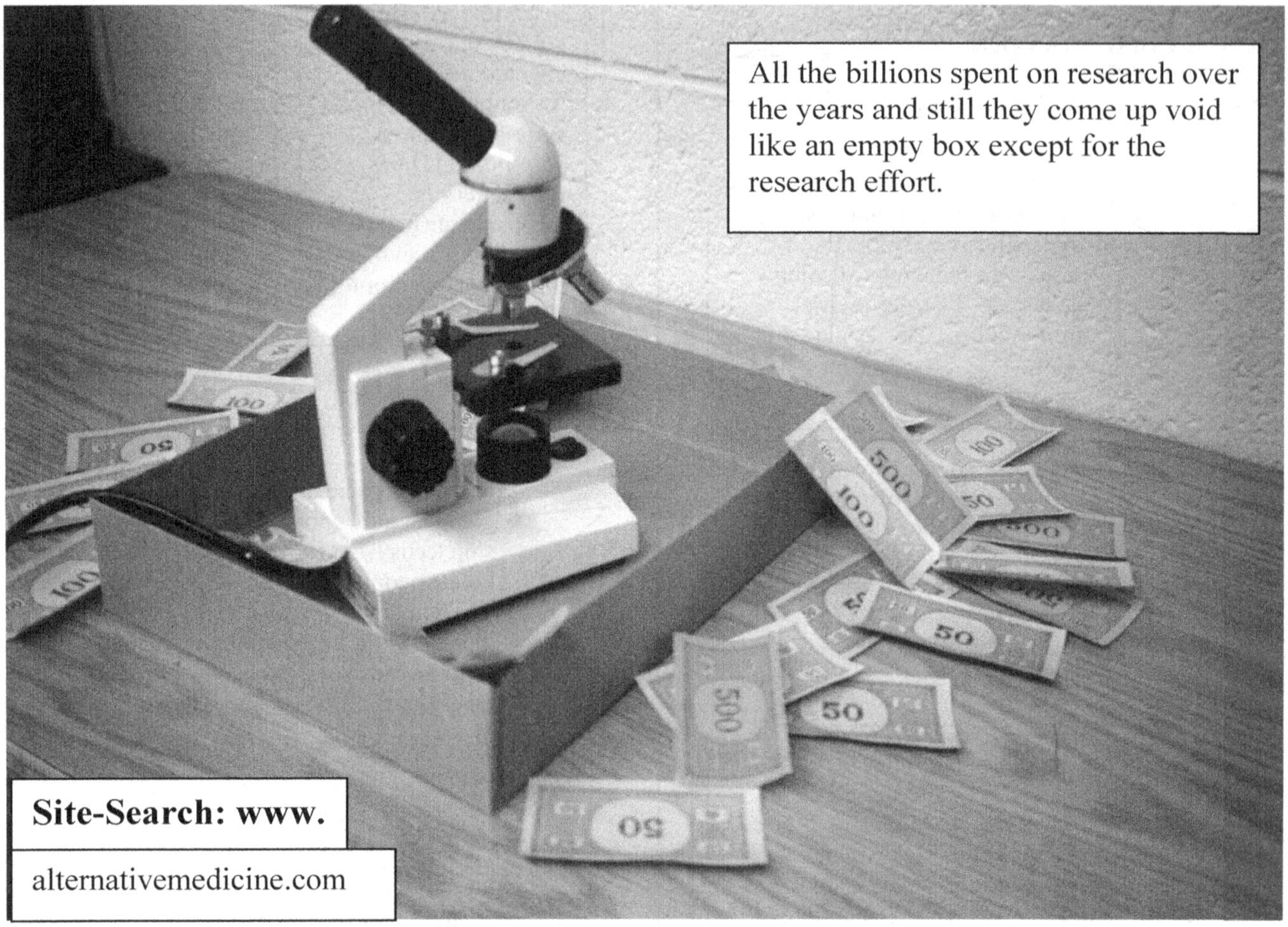

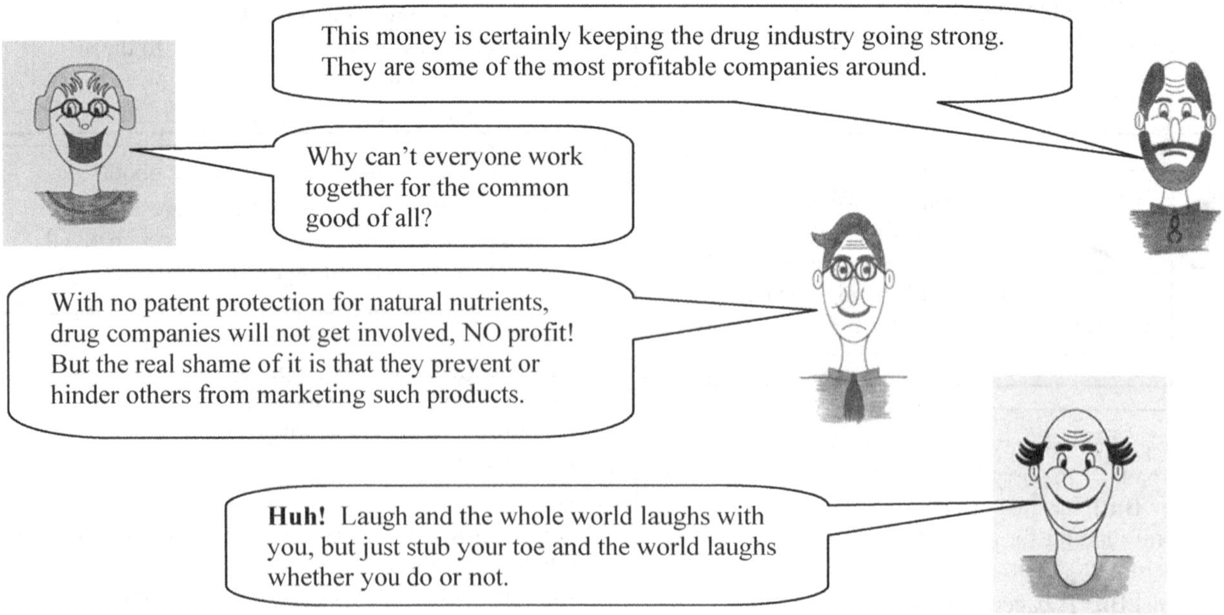

Cancer Crime

Profit before Cure!

Little people pondering?

MITE WORLD©

1

w • Albert, can you imagine that $200 billion has been spent the last 30 years on cancer research with little results? What a crime!

• a Walter, the real crime is that there are cures and treatments for cancer that work and have been denied patients. First, take into account "that half the FDA officials have been formerly employed as key executives in drug companies" [9] and later return to those companies.

2

a • Then little wonder why the FDA suppresses and hinders promotion of alternative options because they are not within the conventional medicine doctrine and profit domain.

• g Is that what the law would call conflict of interest?

• w Apparently not when it comes to billions of **$$** for the drug industry.

3

• g Albert, give some examples.

• g Albert, if I were to get cancer would these options be available to me?

a • Well Gracie, I'll express a few since there are so many options. "Antineoplaston therapy by Dr Burzynski works by having certain amino acids inhibit cancer growth. Shark Cartilage developed by Dr Lane that employs the angiogenesis process, which starves the tumor blood supply. Also Hydrazine Sulfate, which reverses cachexia." [9]

4

a • Yes, Gracie they are available, despite not being sanctioned medical assistance. There is always conventional medicines, surgery, radiation, chemotherapy and the expensive bone morrow transplant that is approved by the FDA, all of which are covered by your health insurance.

w • **Yeah!** That's the cut, burn, poison and near death treatments.

ub • **Sigh!** I quit worrying about my health. It'll go away.

5

• w Albert, since conventional medicine is a big business that has billions of dollars invested in capital equipment, drug research and personnel that require a profitable return, I guess they are protecting themselves?

• a **You bet!** So whenever a new inexpensive holistic substance or procedure appears that can't be patented, there is a knee jerk reaction by the drug companies and the AMA to prevent its utilization.

6

w • I feel like I'm floating down that famous creek without a paddle!

• a Walter, we must be responsible for our own health. With "about 60% of all cancers being related to dietary factors, diet and nutrition are perhaps the most important aspect of any cancer prevention regimen." [9]

Do you know what the difference is between a doctor and God? God does not call himself a doctor.

Happy days are here again!

Celebrate!! I'm free of the big C. The test that drives the nagging fear away.

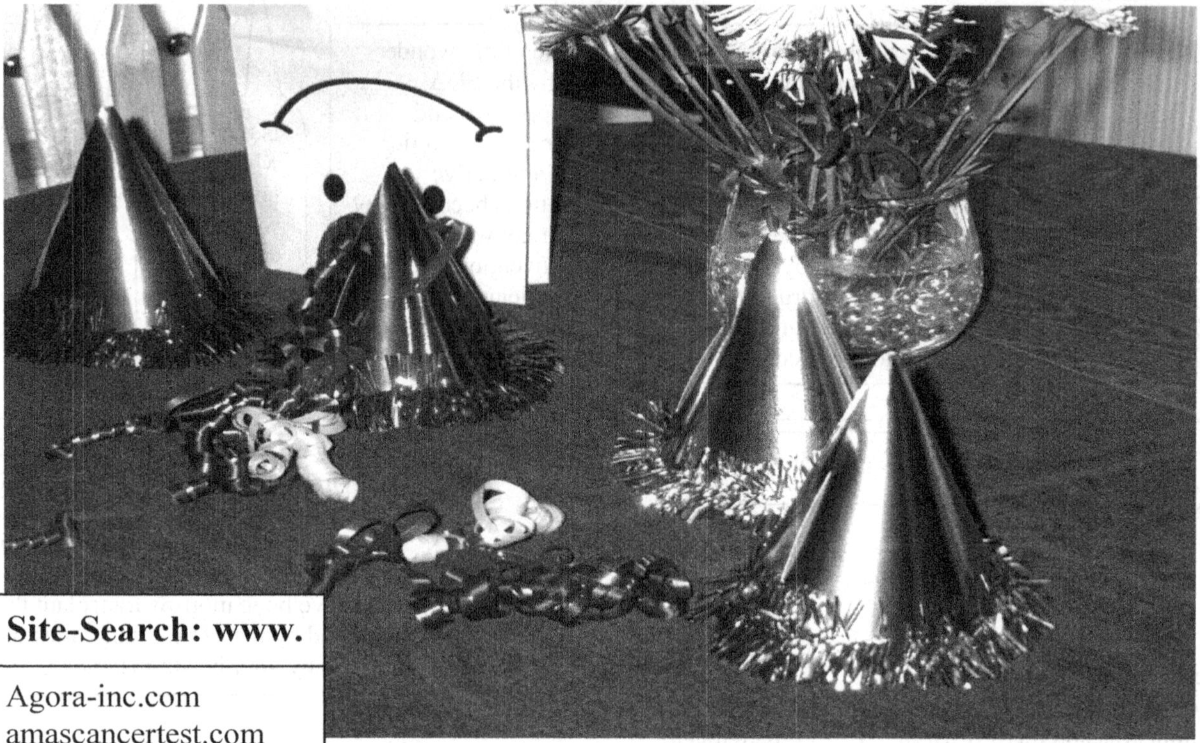

Site-Search: www.

Agora-inc.com
amascancertest.com

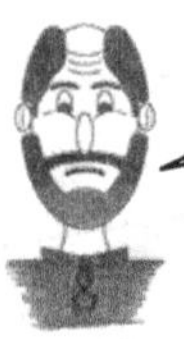

If my doctor is not familiar with this test, what can I do?

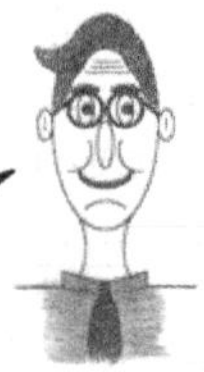

You don't need a doctor's permission to order the AMAS test. "Anyone can order an AMAS test. You receive a free kit in the mail. The kit includes the materials and instructions you need to complete the test, and a packet of scientific literature. Then, take the kit to your doctor or clinic, and ask them to order a blood sample and sign the analysis form. Dr. Bogoch's staff in Boston analyzes all AMAS tests." [11]

Cancer? Not Me! Search, but don't be there!

AMAS early detection test.

1

Little people pondering?

MITE WORLD©

g• Albert, is there some non-invasive way to test to see if one has cancer?

a• Yes Gracie dear, there is an early detection screening method to detect the presence of cancerous cells.

ub• Is this test painful?

2

a• It's only a "simple blood test that can detect precancerous and cancerous cells with up to 99 percent sensitivity." (10)

•w When the nurse is sticking the needle into you Uncle Billy, and she utters that you may feel pressure. **Watch out!** If she says some pressure, **Pow!** You can bet that it'll hurt more. Careful if she says a little pinch. That's a real **Oucher!**

3

•ub I don't think I'll be taking that test.

•a Uncle Billy, Walter is teasing you. This is an inexpensive, relatively painless test with extremely accurate screening results.

•g What is this test called, and what do you mean by early detection screening, Albert?

4

•a It is called the **A**nti- **M**alignin **A**ntibody in **S**erum. This "test can detect the presence of cancerous cells, but can't pinpoint their location. So a positive reading must be followed up by additional testing to locate the cancer and determine its stage." (11)

•ub Maybe now I don't need to spend so much time watching my health with such a test around, and can enjoy life more.

5

w• Is this test good for any kind of cancer, Albert?

•a Yes! "The antibody is manufactured by your own immune system, in response to any kind of cancer cell, which means that one can get treatment before it spreads." (10)

6

•ub I guess it's no longer a question of staying healthy. It's a question of finding a sickness that you like.

a• "Just as important as detection is the monitoring of a disease for the patient after treatment has started." (11)

Do not be like the cat who wanted a fish but was afraid to get his paws wet.
William Shakespeare (1564-1616)

Wring that pain away

Growing old is not for sissies.

Site-Search: www.

drwhitaker.com

hsibaltimore.com

health-pages.com/cgi-local/aff2.pl?SRC=G036T&URL=cy

health.yahoo.com/health/pdr drugs/1829/0.html

life-enhancement.com/displayart.asp?ID=73

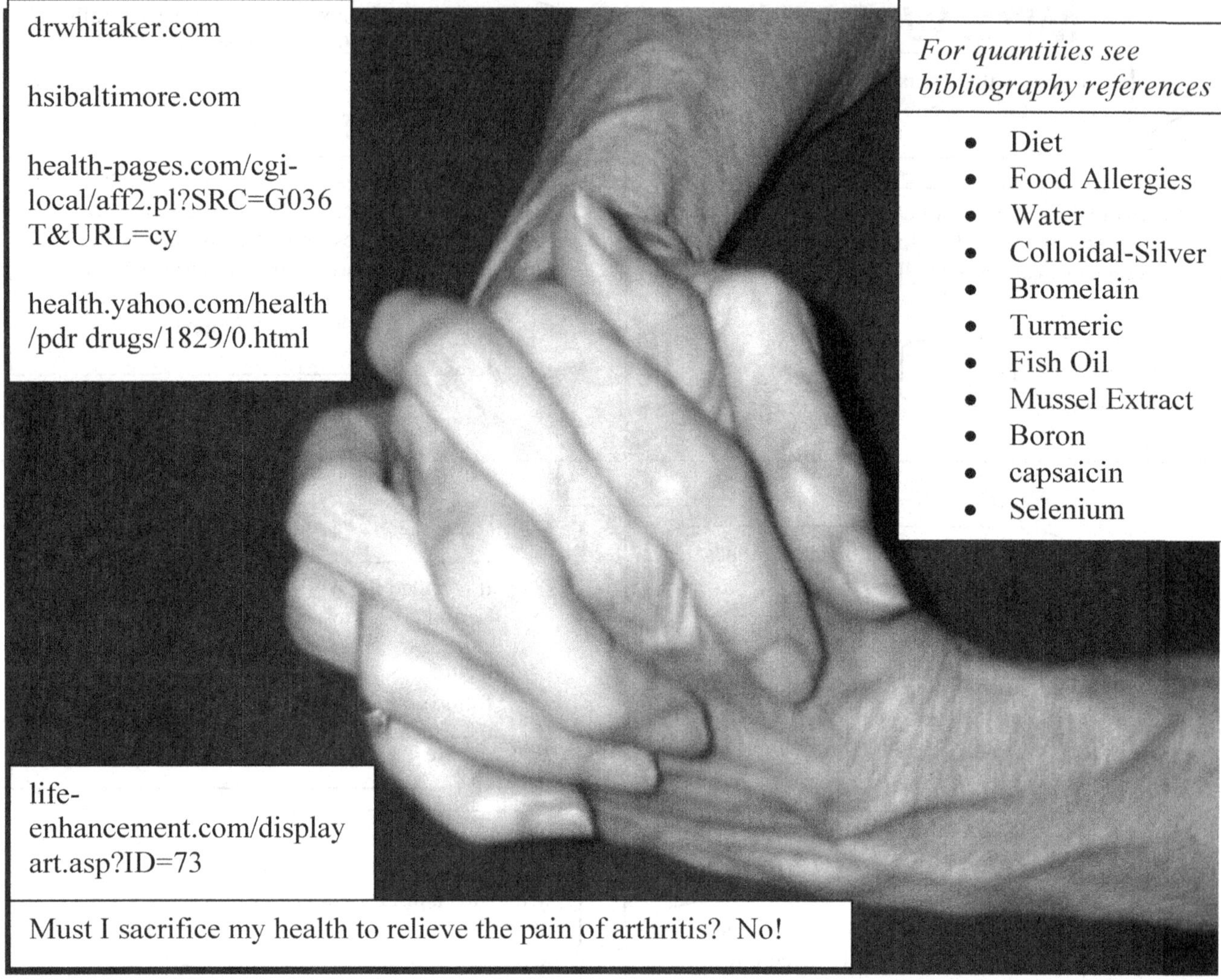

Goodies & Tidbits:

Key search words.

For quantities see bibliography references

- Diet
- Food Allergies
- Water
- Colloidal-Silver
- Bromelain
- Turmeric
- Fish Oil
- Mussel Extract
- Boron
- capsaicin
- Selenium

Must I sacrifice my health to relieve the pain of arthritis? No!

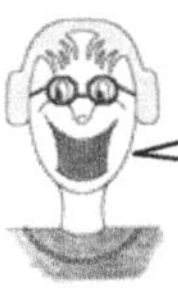

Albert, is there some everyday subtances that I can have my aunt use to relieve arthritis pain?

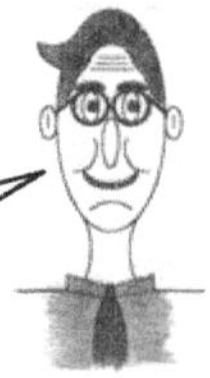

Yes, strange as it may seem Cayenne pepper, the spice from the grocery store, can be used therapeutically to relieve localized pain. "Cayenne pepper has something called capsaicin, which works by depleting substances P a neuropeotide produced by the nerves that carry pain sensation." (12) She "can purchase skin ointments that have capsaicin to relieve arthritis pain." (12)

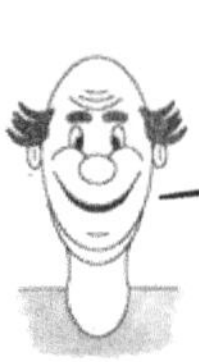

Yipes! Looks like I need to learn more about cooking

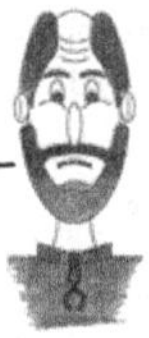

Uncle Billy, you never go into the kitchen except to eat.

Arthritis Living with Pain; Part I

The Symptom called pain

1

Little people pondering?

MITE WORLD©

ub: I see from the title above that this is going to be a long topic. **Prrrettty** important I bet?

g: Albert, my aunt has arthritis and is in terrible pain. The doctor prescribed a NSAID drug to relieve the pain. She is not too happy about taking these drugs after learning that they are "destructive to the joint cartilage and cause kidney failure as well as liver damage." (12) Is there some supplement that she can take to help?

2

ub: I wonder if Sis has to learn to say "**Ow**" in different languages when she travels abroad.

w: **Hmmm..!** There they go again treating the symptom pain and not going for a cure.

a: Well, Gracie dear, this is a difficult problem. Sorry, Walter, there is no cure at this time, but there are several things she can do to help herself. You will be surprised to know that "diet is a major cause of arthritis." (13)

3

w: Can they test for the offending foods?

a: Good point, Walter. The "latest theory is that arthritis is a food allergy. When the body is unable to completely digest the nutrients, the undigested particles are attacked by the immune system causing pain and inflammation. It is difficult to identify the trigger food. The conventional skin prick test is not effective to determine these allergens. A blood test called ALCAT can identify the reacting antibody active in the body. A doctor can have this test done at the AMTL laboratories." (12)

ub: **Food! Foood!** All this talk about food makes me hungry!

4

g: Albert, that was a mouth full. So if she determines what foods she is allergic to and stops eating them will that help her?

a: It will reduce the "symptoms dramatically, also taking a digestive enzyme supplement to help her body properly digest and absorb her food to reduce the effect of the allergies." (13)

w: Is that all there is to it? That's simple enough. What is all the fuss?

a: Believe me, Walter, there is a lot more such as "Mycoplasmas, which are tiny bacteria." (12)

5

a: These "bacteria infect the joints and cause pain and inflammation. Here again is a test PCA-DNA that can detect these creatures." (12)

w: Albert, It's bad enough that you explain everything, but you also explain your explanations. Now I guess you'll tell us what she can do about that?

g: Please do, Albert! What happened to Uncle Billy?

w: I think he went to the kitchen hunting for some food, mumbling something about chicken soup is good for what ails you.

6

a: Success has been experienced using extremely tiny "particle colloidal-silver. Keep in mind not all products are the same. The test conducted used colloidal-silver that was 3-5 parts /million. Being so small reduces toxicity." (12) She also could "start taking selenium, zinc and fish oil for the omega-3 fatty acids to reduce the tenderness in the joints. Boron eases the pain and restores flexibility." (13) Back so soon Uncle Billy? Finished the soup?

ub: **Yeah**, and corn bread, I'm stuffed. Are you done with this part? Can I turn the page now to continue?

Build up those joints

Attacking the problem best way to drive the pain away

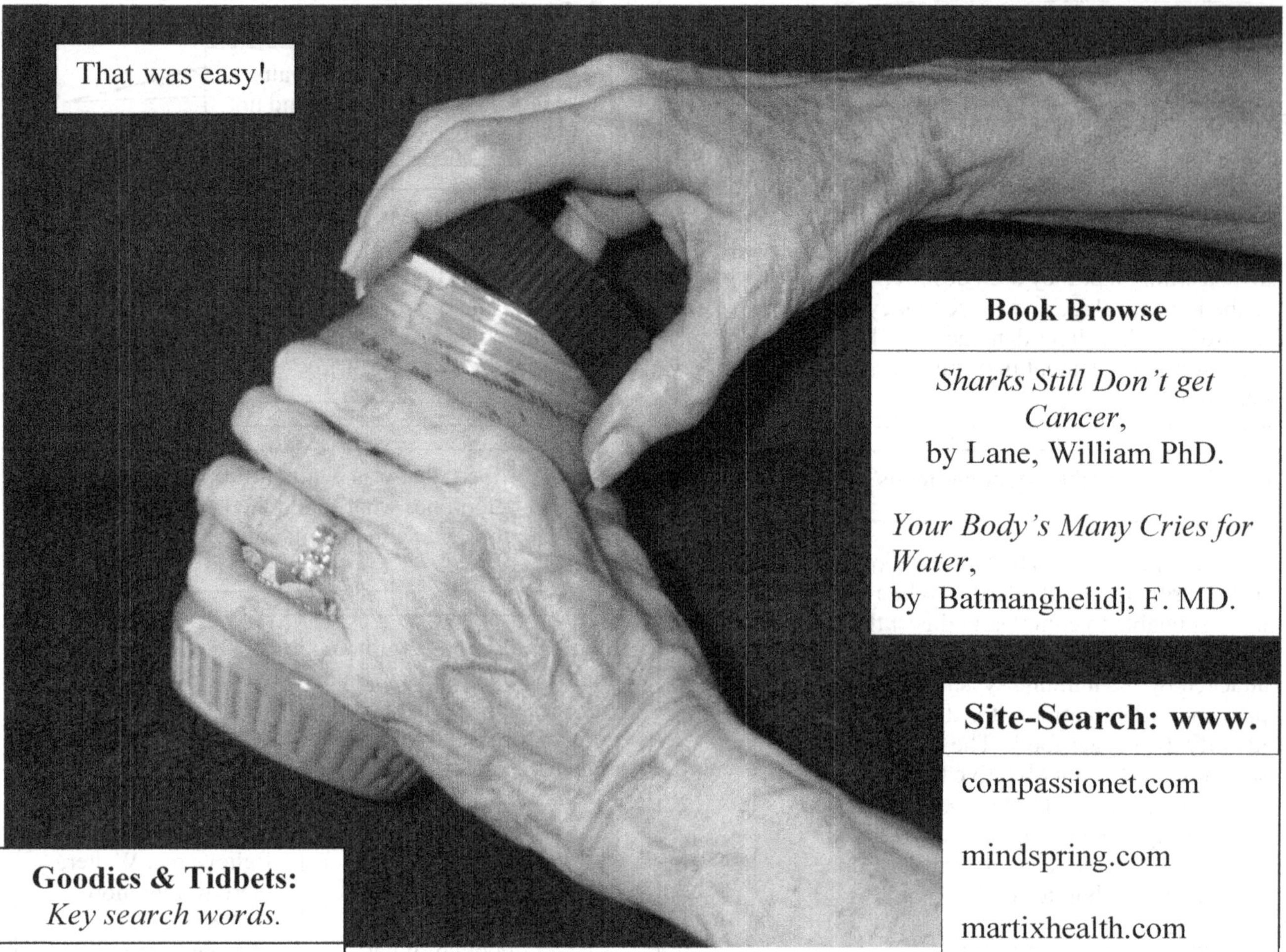

Book Browse

Sharks Still Don't get Cancer, by Lane, William PhD.

Your Body's Many Cries for Water, by Batmanghelidj, F. MD.

Site-Search: www.

compassionet.com

mindspring.com

martixhealth.com

watercure.com

hsibaltimore.com

drwhitaker.com

Goodies & Tidbets:
Key search words.

For quantities see bibliography references

- Glucosamine
- Chondroitin
- Shark Cartilage
- Fish Oil
- Green Mussel Extract
- Water

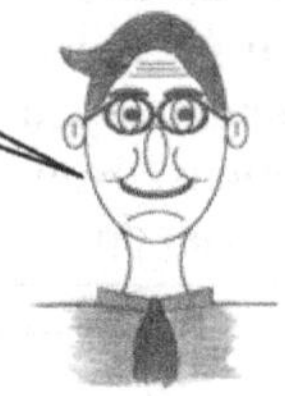

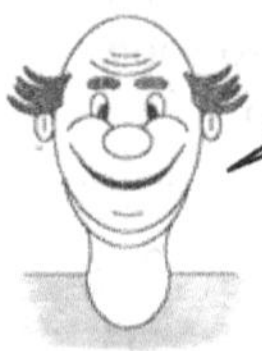

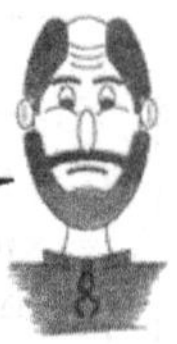

Arthritis Repair Part II

More than Treating Symptoms.

1

Little people pondering?

MITE WORLD©

w: I read that glucosamine and chondroitin are helpful in rebuilding joint cartilage.

ub: Glucosamine sounds like a racehorse I once bet on and lost my shirt, it was called gluepotsamighty.

a: Correct Walter, "glucosamine and chondroitin sulfate supplements help the body repair damaged joints while attracting water to the cartilage, which is important." [13]

2

a: Another "problem with NSAID's is that they block the body's ability to heal itself and accelerate the joint damage even though there is short term pain relief." [13]

g: Albert, my aunt heard that shark cartilage is beneficial to joint repair.

a: It has been "documented so. Shark cartilage has natural glucosamine and chondroitin." [12] **Alsoo….**

3

ub: **Oh-boy!** Those sharks better watch out now. People will fish sharks to extinction for their cartilage.

w: **Ex-cccuse me** Uncle Billy, Albert please continue.

a: "It has certain proteins that prevent additional blood-vessel invasion of the joints and collagen that improves the efficacy in treating arthritis." [12]

4

g: I guess auntie can go right out and buy some cartilage.

a: Careful, not all cartilage is the same. I generally don't specify a brand, but in this case I suggest only "Benefin for its production purity and test record. Also, it comes in an ointment as well as a supplement." [12]

ub: I guess now-a-days the only way to keep your health is to eat what you don't want, drink what you don't like and do what ever you'd rather not.

5

w: Are there other things one can do for arthritis, Albert?

a: There are a number of different nutrients that have anti-inflammatory and pain relief properties.

ub: Don't get carried away, Albert.

6

a: First, there is "MSM to help against inflammation." [12] Simple as it may sound, it is very helpful to "drink water to keep your joints hydrated." [12] There are other herbs also. Short enough, Uncle Billy?

ub: **Gee thanks!** Albert. I know filtered water of course.

ub: **Sigh! All done!**

"Man is in constant **repair**", we must continually nourish ourselves to maintain a strong immune system. *Samuel Johnson 1709-1784*

Water

body & soul

Prayer cleanses the soul
Water cleanses the body
The first requires a pure heart
The other requires no impurities.

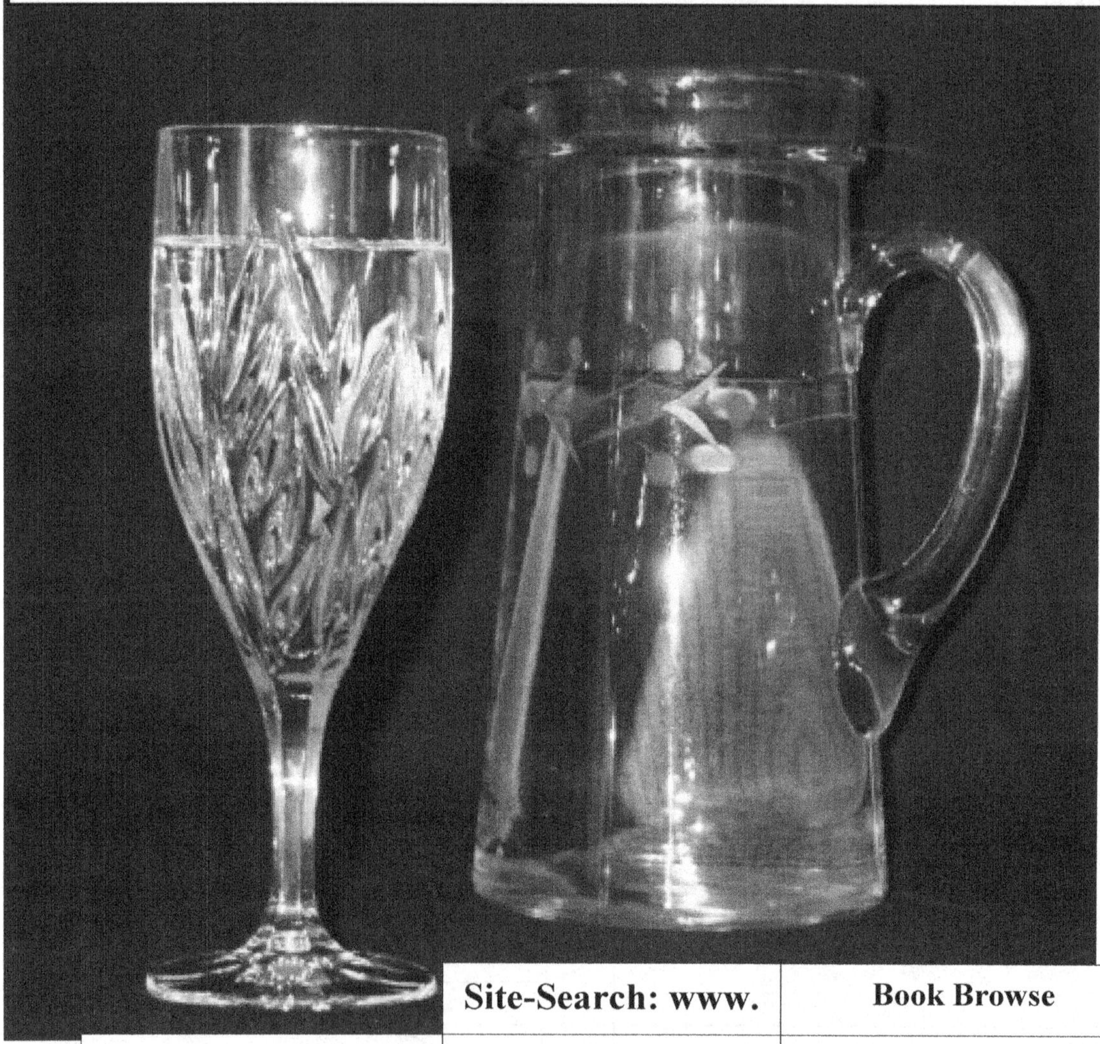

Site-Search: www.
Watercure.com

Book Browse
Your Body's Many Cries for Water by Batmanghelidj, F. MD.

Goodies & Tidbits: *Key Words*
• Filtered Water • Dehydration

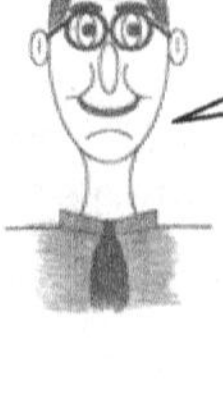

"Tea, coffee, alcohol and manufactured beverages such as sodas are no substitutes for water. This is a self-imposed restriction on the water needs of the body, which can lead to dehydration and in turn to disease conditions." (14)

Dehydration the origin of much Infirmity

Water! Water everywhere except the body!

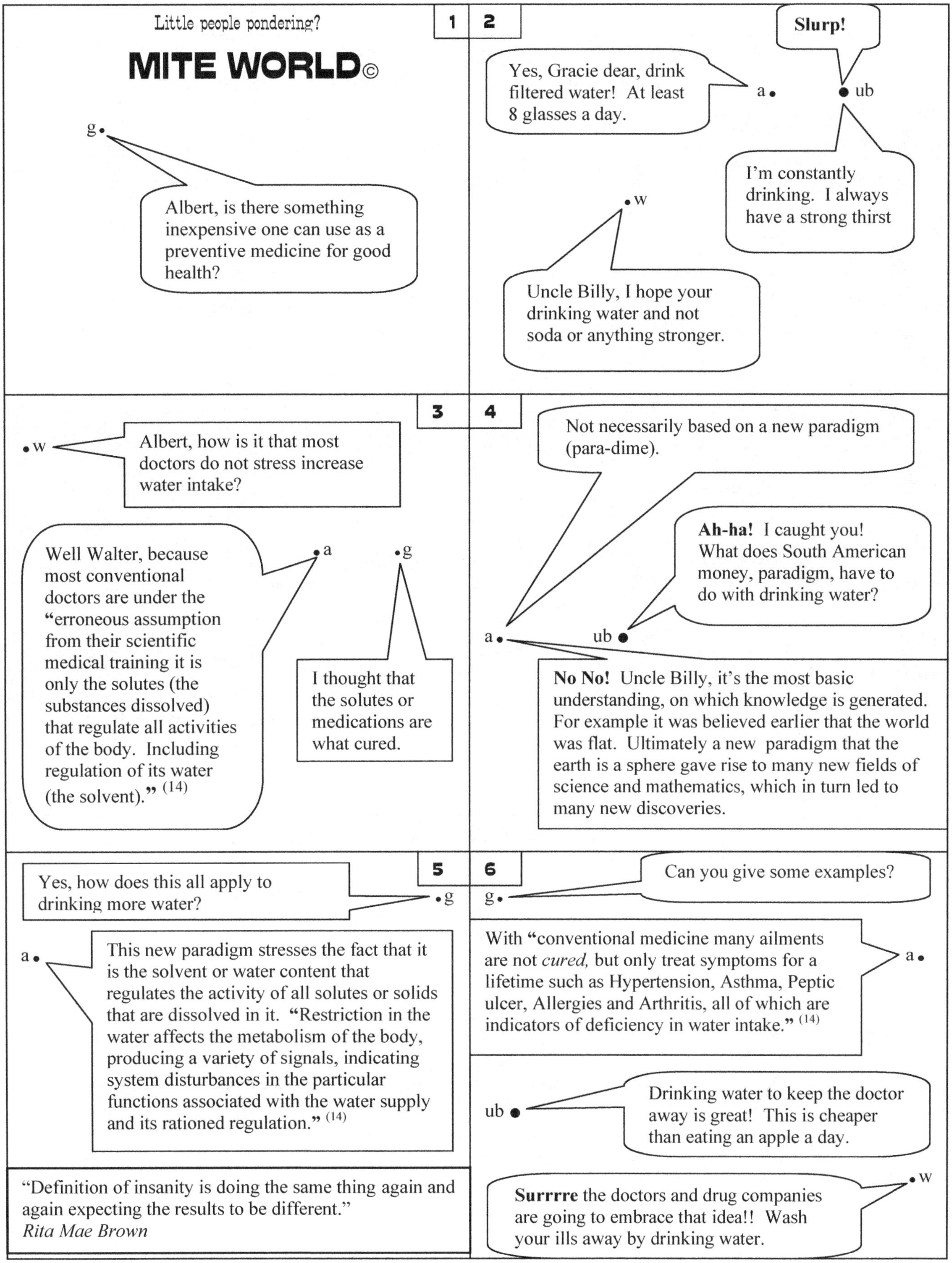

Inhale, Exhale

Getting the Power of Oxygen

The world is so unfair. Why do the rich people have all the money? Still you can breathe the same air at the same price. Hopefully this is without pollution.

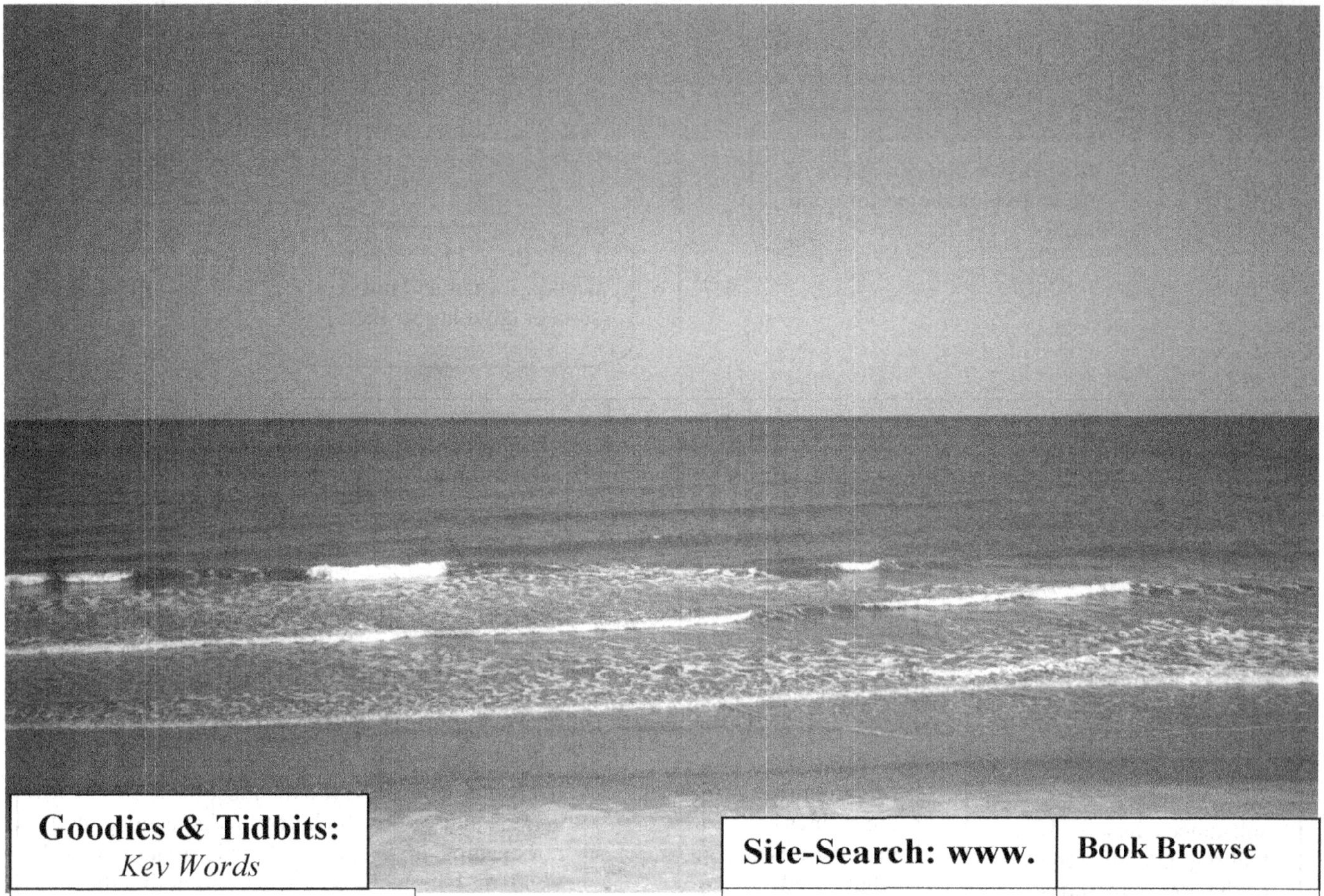

Goodies & Tidbits:
Key Words

- Diet
- Exercise
- Power Walking
- Aerobatic Breathing

Site-Search: www.	**Book Browse**
oxycise.com	*Oxycise* by Johnson, Jill

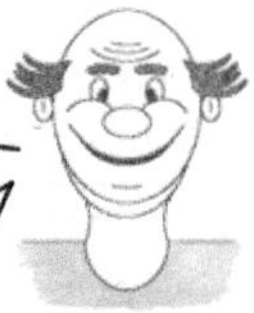

I've been breathing fine all my life and I'm still here.

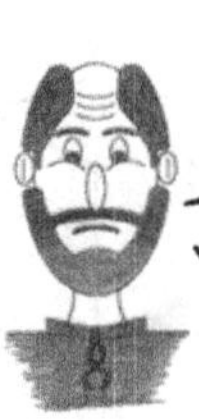

Yeah! A whole bunch of you, Uncle Billy.

Aaugh! I don't need a perfect body; I've had this one for so long, I've grown attached to it. Sounds like I need to go to college to learn to breathe proper.

I'm glad you never let schooling interfere with your education, Uncle Billy.

Breathing takes practice for Wellness & Weight loss

Suck in that Oxygen

Little people pondering?

MITE WORLD©

1

g: Albert is there something else that I can do for my wellness that is inexpensive and easy?

ub: **Yeah!** With emphasis on easy.

a: Most definitely, the very air that we breathe, Gracie dear. This is the exception where conventional and holistic medicine agrees. Exercise particularly aerobic exercise.

2

ub: **Aaugh!** I knew that there was a catch somewhere. **Aerobic!**

g: Quiet, Uncle Billy, go ahead Albert.

w: Doctors exercise. They get to play their Wednesday golf, without a golf cart. Maybe?

a: Believe it or not, walking is one of the best forms of exercise. No jolting or impacting like jogging. No heavy weights to lift that strain the muscles. Best of all, no expensive equipment or gym fees. You can walk just by going out the front door.

3

w: Albert, you stressed aerobic exercise. You don't mean a stroll.

a: It's certainly not the best, but it's better than lounging in front of a TV munching snacks. It's important to get your body in motion and breathe correctly.

ub: I breathe just fine, I'm pushing 80- that's enough exercise for me.

g: Albert, how do you recommend to walk for exercise?

4

a: Take a brisk walk at least 3 times a week. Walk a distance of 2 miles, that's 1 mile from your home and back. This should be done in a half hour. If you do this you're walking at a 4mile/hour rate, which is called power walking.

ub: Where does the breathing part come in?

a: Most people are "shallow chest breathers. This is poor ventilation of their lungs. Putting their body in an anaerobic state setting themselves up for a host of disorders from skin problems to heart disease, cancer and obesity." [15]

5

w: **Phew!** Enough already. How should I breathe for wellness?

ub: **Yeah!** I agree.

g: **Hush!** Guys

a: Its called "diaphragmatic breathing." [15] Use your diaphragm to breath. Extend your stomach and inhale oxygen through your nose. Exhale carbon dioxide through the mouth. Breathe this way while you're walking or working around the house.

6

g: Albert, you said that this would help with weight lost?

a: Try the "Oxycise System." [15] It's a breathing and stretching technique to help lose weight that is done at home. "studies have shown that this is as effective as a stationary bike." [15]

"All parts of the body which have function, if used in moderation and exercised in labors in which each is accustomed, become thereby healthy, well-developed and age more slowly, but if unused they become liable to disease, defective in growth, and age quickly."
Hippocrates

Brainwashing. I wonder if they have some doubts about their product?

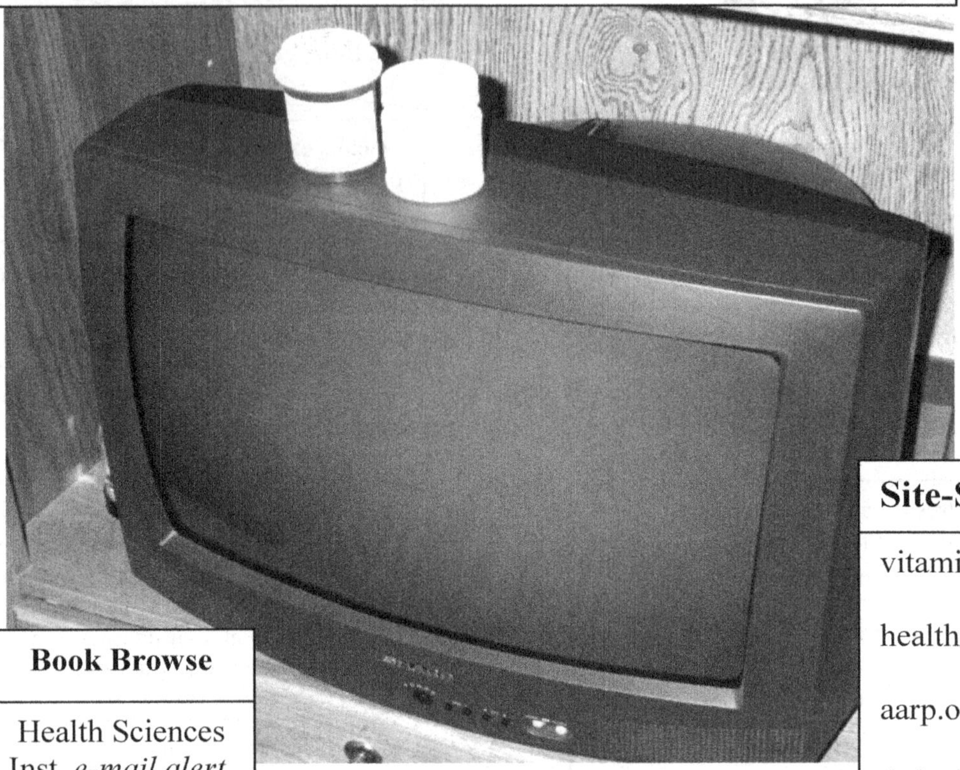

Book Browse

Health Sciences Inst. *e-mail alert,* May 2002

Site-Search: www.

vitamins-for-all.org

healthchoice.org.uk

aarp.org/bulletin

drdavidwilliams.com

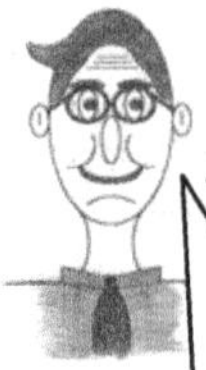

The pharmaceutical companies are hurting from the Holistic enterprises biting into their profits that they are now lobbying the legislation to pass laws, which would classify natural nutrients as medical drugs rather than food supplements, thereby requiring a doctor's prescription. It's like they're passing a law against prevention.

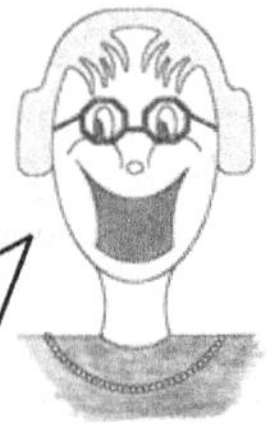

Sounds like these big druggy companies want complete control of everything for more profits in their pockets. It certainly doesn't look like they believe in free enterprise to me.

"Not only are the drug companies eliminating competition from natural products for treating illnesses, they are essentially forcing greater need for prescription products. After all, without prevention, where will people be forced to turn when they get even the slightest bit ill; to physicians who will prescribe mainstream pharmaceuticals or super-strength, prescription-only vitamins. Supplied by - **guess who** - the big international pharmaceutical companies." (16)

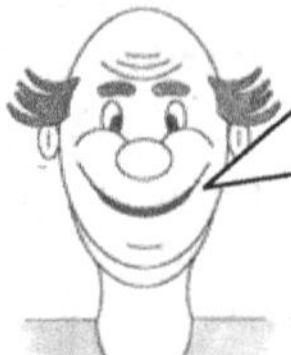

They say that "Justice is blind," but you have to wonder if she shouldn't have developed a better sense of smell. Because this stinks!

Advertising Prescription Drugs on TV.

Pester your doctor for those drugs!

Little people pondering?

MITE WORLD©

1

g: Albert, if the drug is advertised on TV it must be OK?

a: Maybe, Gracie dear, many drugs are approved by the FDA then withdrawn. In 1997 the FDA approved pharmaceutical companies to advertise prescription drugs.

2

a: "Marketers know that the more familiar a product is the less intimidating and frightening it becomes the more acceptable and profitable." (16)

w: **Sigh!** How is it that opportunity knocks once, but TV drug commercials swamp us repeatedly every night?

3

a: Aggressive promotion of drugs to the consumer and doctors alike all help to sell drugs. "This kind of advertising is banned in nearly all other Western countries. The drug companies spent $2.5 billion/year on mass media advertising," (17) which contributes to drug cost.

w: Drug prices are rising twice the rate of inflation.

ub: **Yeah!** My doctor gives me free samples when I start a new prescription. How can he do that?

4

a: Uncle Billy, the drug companies give doctors "$8 billion /year free samples to promote products." (17) They "employ 87,000 marketing representatives" (17) to do this promotion. Not only to give free samples, but gifts such as paid vacations. Again pushing the drug sale & cost to us **Up Up & Away**.

g: I would think that doctors could lose their objectivity.

w: Since most of the drugs are very similar, huge advertising campaigns are needed much like any household detergent.

5

g: Albert, the TV advertisements are pleasant and very attractive.

a: Very professionally done Gracie, but as you watch the healthy people prance about in the beautiful ocean or farm field vista, listen to the commentator describe all the side effects.

g: I must admit that I do get distracted. Albert, many of these drugs are very popular.

6

a: A lot of people are looking for instant relief, Gracie. Keep in mind that many drugs treat the symptoms, but do not cure the ailment.

ub: **Groan!** I hope I'm sick!
I hope I'm sick!
I hope I'm sick!

a: Why do you want to be sick, Uncle Billy?

ub: Well I'd hate to be well and feel like this.

The best way for a doctor to prevent a malpractice is to cure the patient!

"I'm concerned because today there are so many hazards to health, so many toxins to beware of, and so great a need to be vigilant to keep your health in top form. Here are some health tips for my grandchildren and all the children in this country as they enter adulthood:" quoted from Dr. Burton Goldberg, see his "*A Health letter to my grandchildren*" at his web site. .www.alternativemedicine.com/AMHome.asp?cn=Catalog&act=GetProduct&crt=ProductKey=9689&Style=/AMXSL/EssayDetail.xsl

It is interesting that everyone asserts their love and concern for their children yet almost every school day most send them off to school in school buses without seat belts! We need to be informed about the alternative options for good health that are available, so as not to send them out into the world without a wellness seat belt for protection. Just a pondering?

Sunlight – Let the real light in.

Lest we forget that the eyes are the gateway to the mind

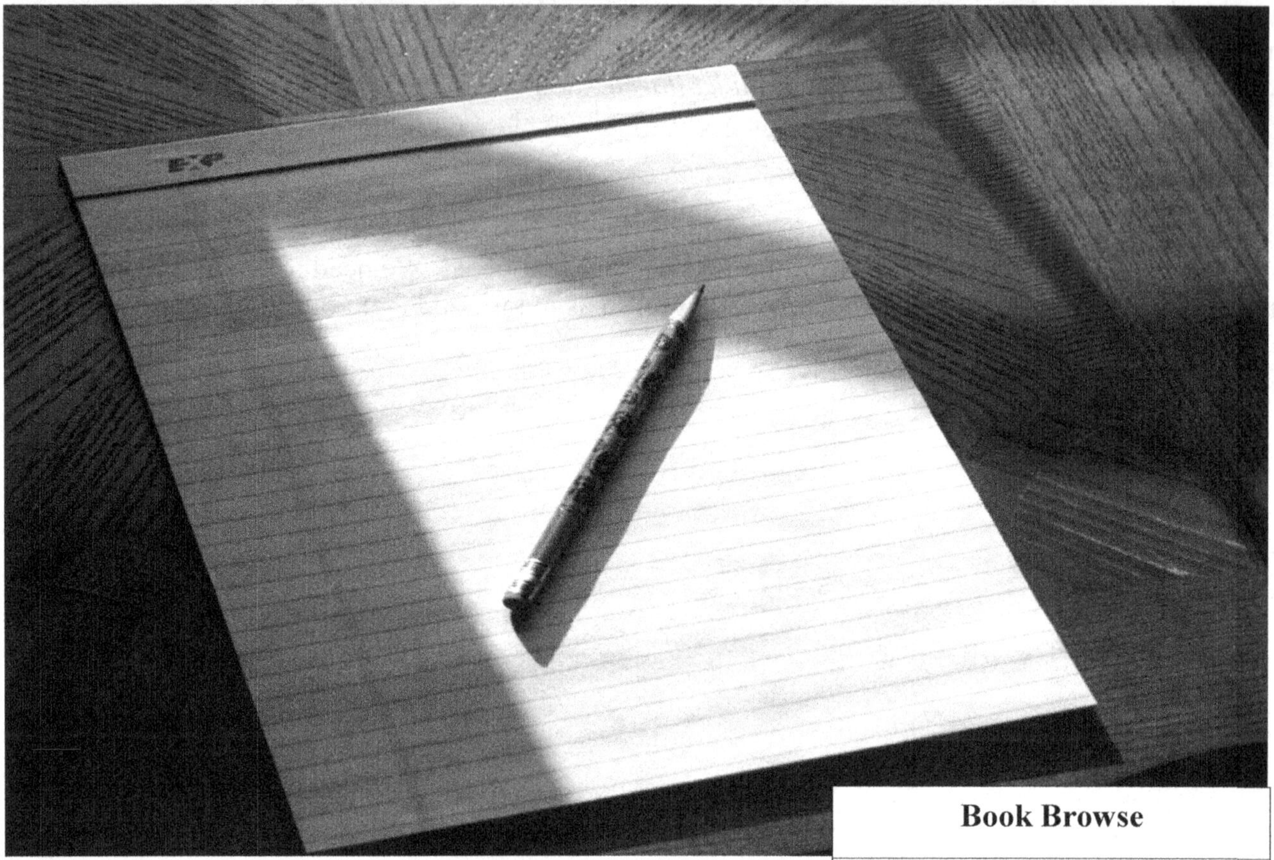

Book Browse

Into the Light.
by Douglass, W. C. MD.

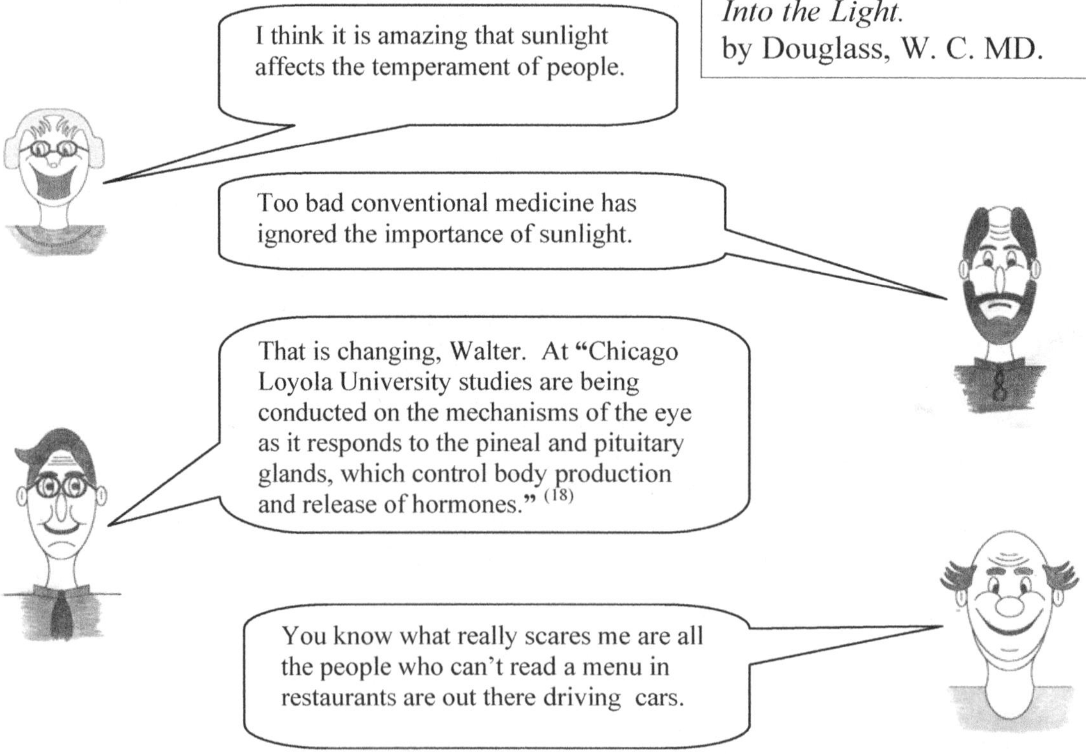

Student Hyperactivity & Fluorescent Light.

Let there be sunlight.

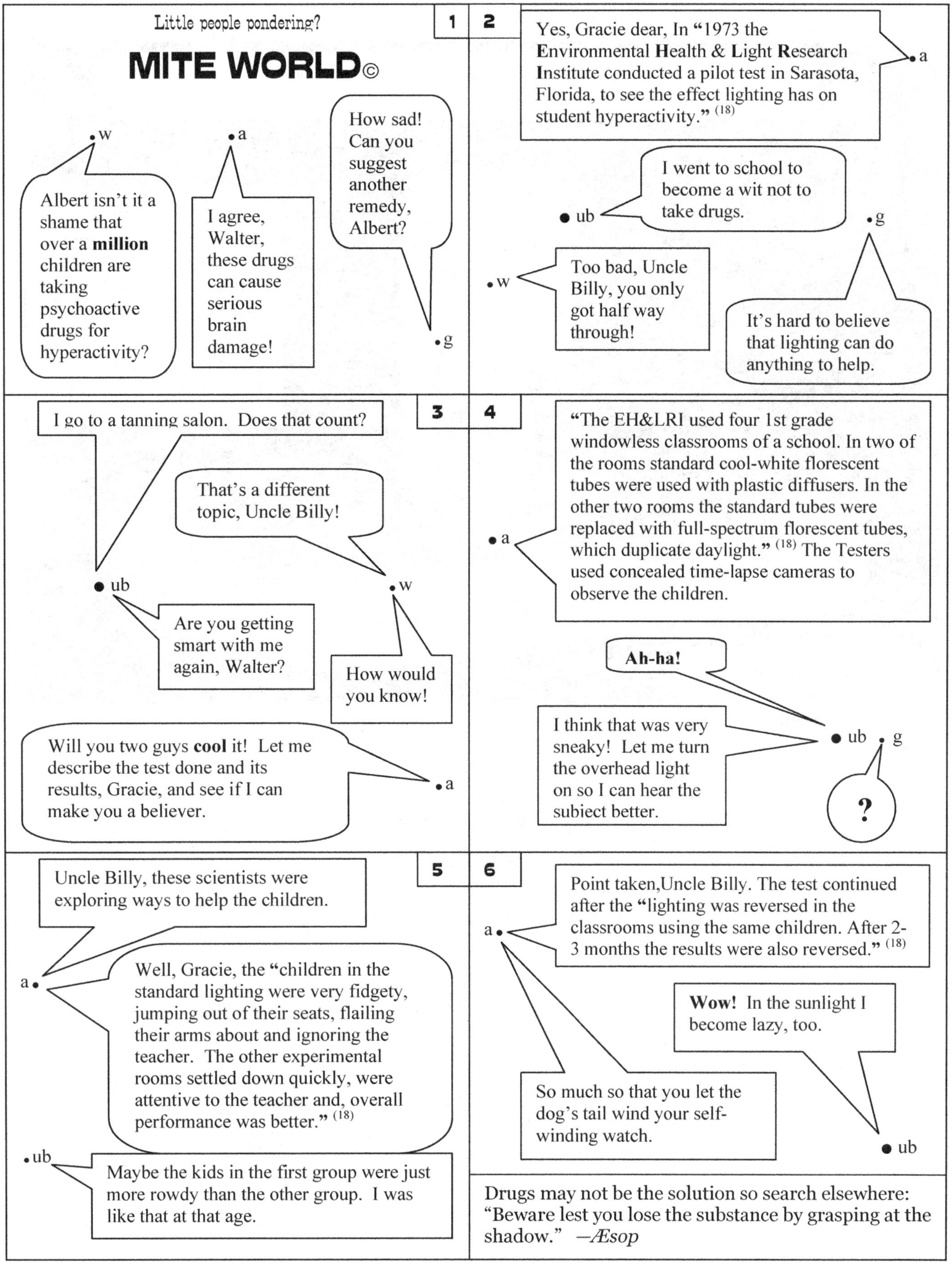

Don't mix well- food???

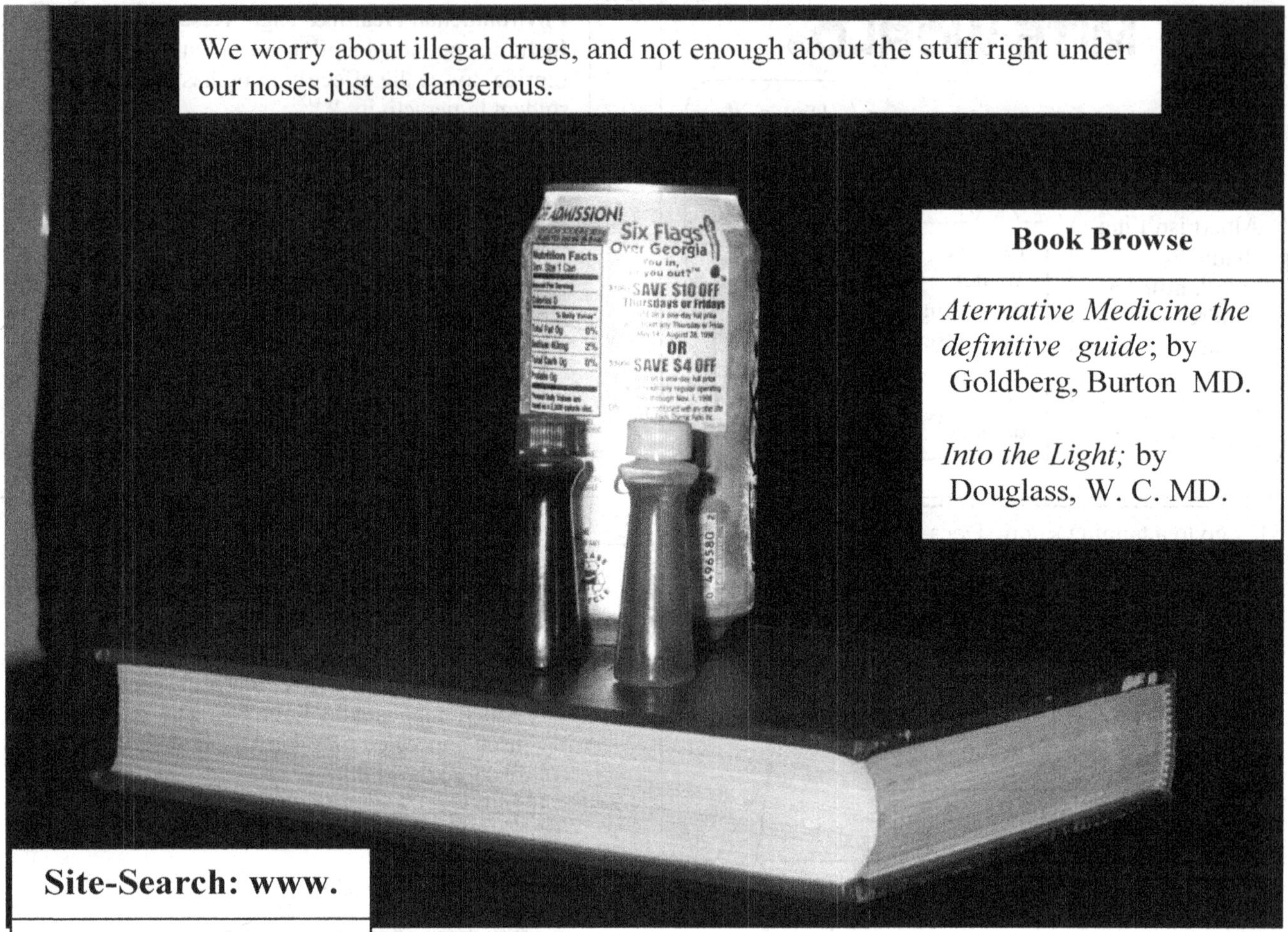

We worry about illegal drugs, and not enough about the stuff right under our noses just as dangerous.

Book Browse

Aternative Medicine the definitive guide; by Goldberg, Burton MD.

Into the Light; by Douglass, W. C. MD.

Site-Search: www.

alternativemedicine.com

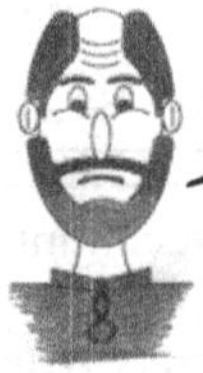

It seems like the everyday things taken for granted had a big impact on all of us, such as the food we eat, drink and even the light we are exposed to.

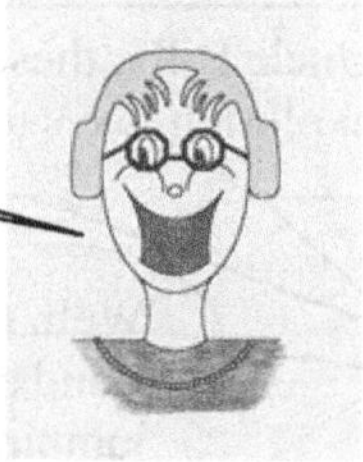

Particularly with children.

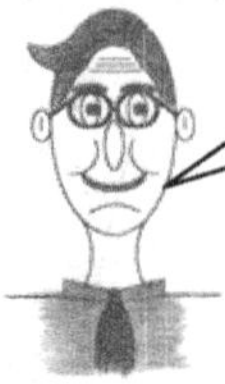

Studies have been done relating the interaction between fluorescent lighting and artificial food coloring. It is similar to an allergic reaction manifested as hyperactivity in children.

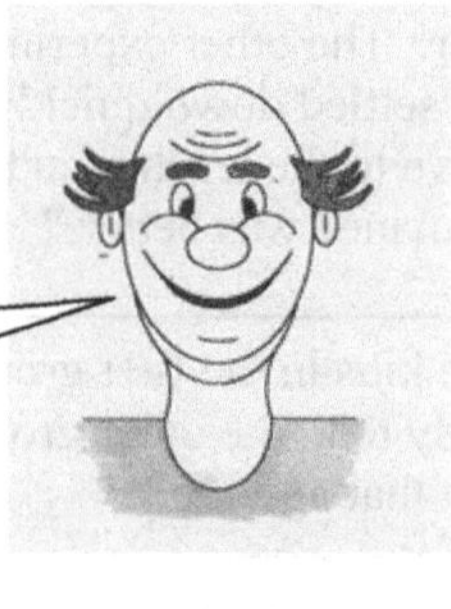

I was hyperactive as a kid. Maybe that was because I was a light eater. As soon as it got light I started to eat.

The Food Industry Harms our Children's Education.

Purge food additives.

1

Little people pondering?

MITE WORLD©

•g Albert, is it true that diet effects children's learning ability and attention span?

•a Yes, Gracie dear, to explain, I may bore you with some history.

2

•w Please continue, Albert, but give us the abbreviated version.

• ub Go ahead. As long as I can rest on the couch while you talk. Please, keep it short. History is boring!

Maybe, Uncle Billy, you can get a job as a tester in a mattress factory?

Where do you think I work now?

3

•a You bet Walter, the effects of diet on learning begins in "1979 New York City public schools ranked in the 39th percentile on the Scholastic Achievement Test Scores. That year the NYC Board of Education ordered a reduction of the sugar content of foods served in the schools and banned two synthetic food colorings. In 1980 the SATS went up to the 47th percentile. Next the schools banned all synthetic food colorings. The following year the scores increased to the 51st percentile." [19]

• ub ZZZZZZZZZZZZ ZZZZZZ!

4

•w Uncle Billy, you're snoring too loud. Remeber that there is going to be a test after.

•a I'm afraid that the only cure for Uncle Billy is insomnia. "By 1983 the schools next removed the food additives BHA & BHT. You know what? The scores again increased, to the 55th percentile. Prior to the dietary changes the scores never varied more than 1% in a year's time." [19]

Ho-hum!

• ub I'm awake, Walter! Albert is done, **Amen**! He sure was on a roll. Does that mean that if those changes were made when I went to school I wouldn't have been able to drink soda?

5

•g Yes, Uncle Billy! Albert, I would think that the schools would need a trained dietitian to set-up menus and substitute different foods, which all will cost more money than the schools would want to spend.

•a An excellent point, Gracie, since schools are federally mandated and subsidized to feed the students there is a budget in place. Changing to the correct diet may be the more controversial issue. This is well-spent money.

Youth comes, but once with the opportunity to learn. "Do not squander time for that is the stuff that life is made of." - *Ben Franklin (1706-1790)*

6

•g Why don't other schools adopt this diet plan? Also, I'm concerned that the children wouldn't eat the healthier food, but just dump it in the garbage pail!

•a The educational systems are very bureaucratic, conventional and generally not open to methods outside their realm. It's true that adjustments are needed.

I guess what we eat is what we are. Too bad I didn't eat right when I was young.

• ub

•w Too bad you didn't take a history pill back then.

It was too big to swallow.

Teens & Antidepressants can = guns.

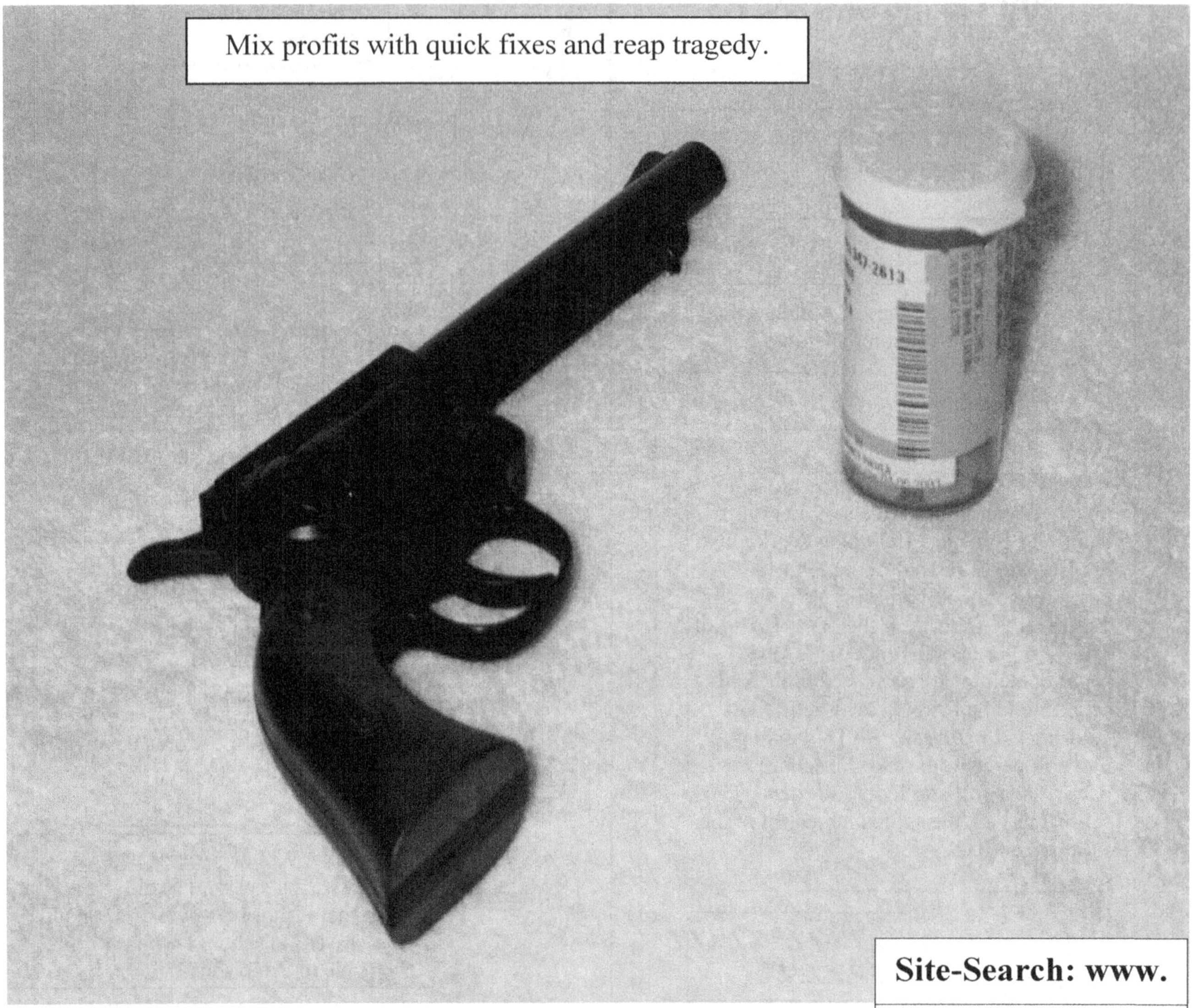

Site-Search: www.

drwhitaker.com

discover.com

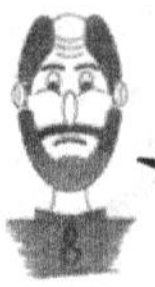

This country has become so drug orientated that **"**doctors are now prescribing SSRI's to 3-5 year old children using the new designation ODD, **O**ppositional **D**efiant **D**isorder as the excuse**"** (21)

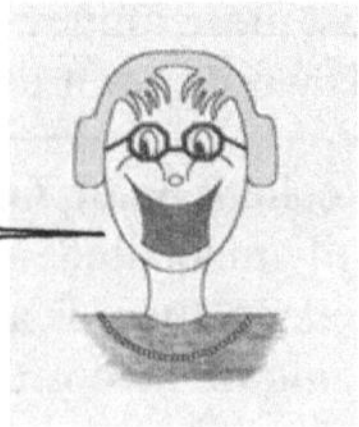

How frightening!

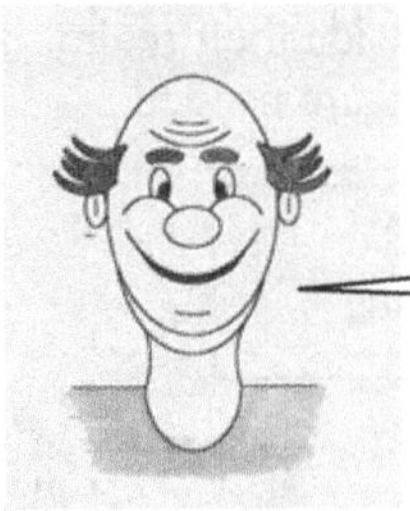

I guess I can go to school now, act up and get drugs to get high?

Teenage Violence & Antidepressant (SSRI's)

What do Luvox and Columbine have in common?

Little people pondering?

MITE WORLD ©

1

•g Albert, isn't it terrible about the teenage shootings? This must be due to the accessibility of guns and the media's glamorization of violence.

a• It doesn't help, Gracie dear. Did you know that "Eric Harris, one of the Columbine killers, was on the anti-depressant Luvox."?[21]

2

•a Also, an "Oregon teen, Kip Kinkel after killing his parents, went on a rampage killing 2 and wounding 22 of his fellow students at Thurston High. He had been taking Prozac." [21]

•g **No!** The media was quiet about SSRI's

•w I read that it was "recognized from the beginning that the side effects included violent impulses, agitation and sexual dysfunction." [20]

3

•g Albert, at the school where I work, a lot of the kids are on Ritalin.

a• Sorry to hear that, Gracie, It's a quick fix to manage the excitable children, but it could have a stiff price someday. Young brains still maturing need proper nourishment. Not antidepressants that only upset the brain chemistry more and mask the symptoms of the real problem. Good diet would be of more value to the victimizer as well as the victims.

4

• ub I knew a man who was a paranoid schizophrenic and always thought he was following himself.

•w Uncle Billy, I never knew that you knew such big words?

• ub **Ah-ha!** I was told this story and liked it, so I memorized it. Don't ask me to explain what I said.

•a When Walter was a young boy our parents didn't give him drugs, they pleaded with him to just run away.

5

g• Albert, these stories you're quoting must be exceptional?

•w **Whoa!** Albert thanks for your endorsement! Gracie, these drugs are all legal not stuff being imported from Columbia, but from USA drug companies.

a• I'm afraid not. Gracie. Another example is about a "teen in Ft. Gibson, Oklahoma that started shouting "I'm crazy!" over and over again then emptied his gun shooting 5 of his classmates. He was on SSRI's" [21]

6

g• I understand that Prozac is one of the most successful drugs ever with huge revenues.

•a My concern is the "30 million Americans taking this type drug where there is no consensus on how they truly work." [20]

•w I have a friend who went to a psychiatrist for depression and told him that he had suicidal tendencies. The doctor prescribed Prozac and said that from now on he had to pay in advance.

"Measure a thousand times and cut once." (*Turkish Proverb*). A child's mind is a precious thing. Don't temper with it casually, and create an irreversible condition. Proceed cautiously.

ENVIRONMENT

In the months to come we will be hearing more and more about the nation's electricity being generated from *renewable resources* using the **R**enewable **P**ortfolio **S**tandards (RPS). This energy and energy efficiency policies will be enacted in the states as proposed at the federal level. These policies will formulate renewable energy funds, which could be used to lower the costs and encourage the development of emerging technologies like photovoltaic, fuel cells, wind and solar thermal power.

Replacing fossil fuels with renewables would help provide considerable environmental benefits as well as reduced dependence on foreign oil. The United States would reduce CO_2 and other pollutants that harm the environment and human health. We need to keep ourselves informed to respond to our elected officials to keep them on track. Just a pondering?

Power- the good & the bad

Energy-Yes Pollution- No!

Cloning power plants like this the only answer? No!

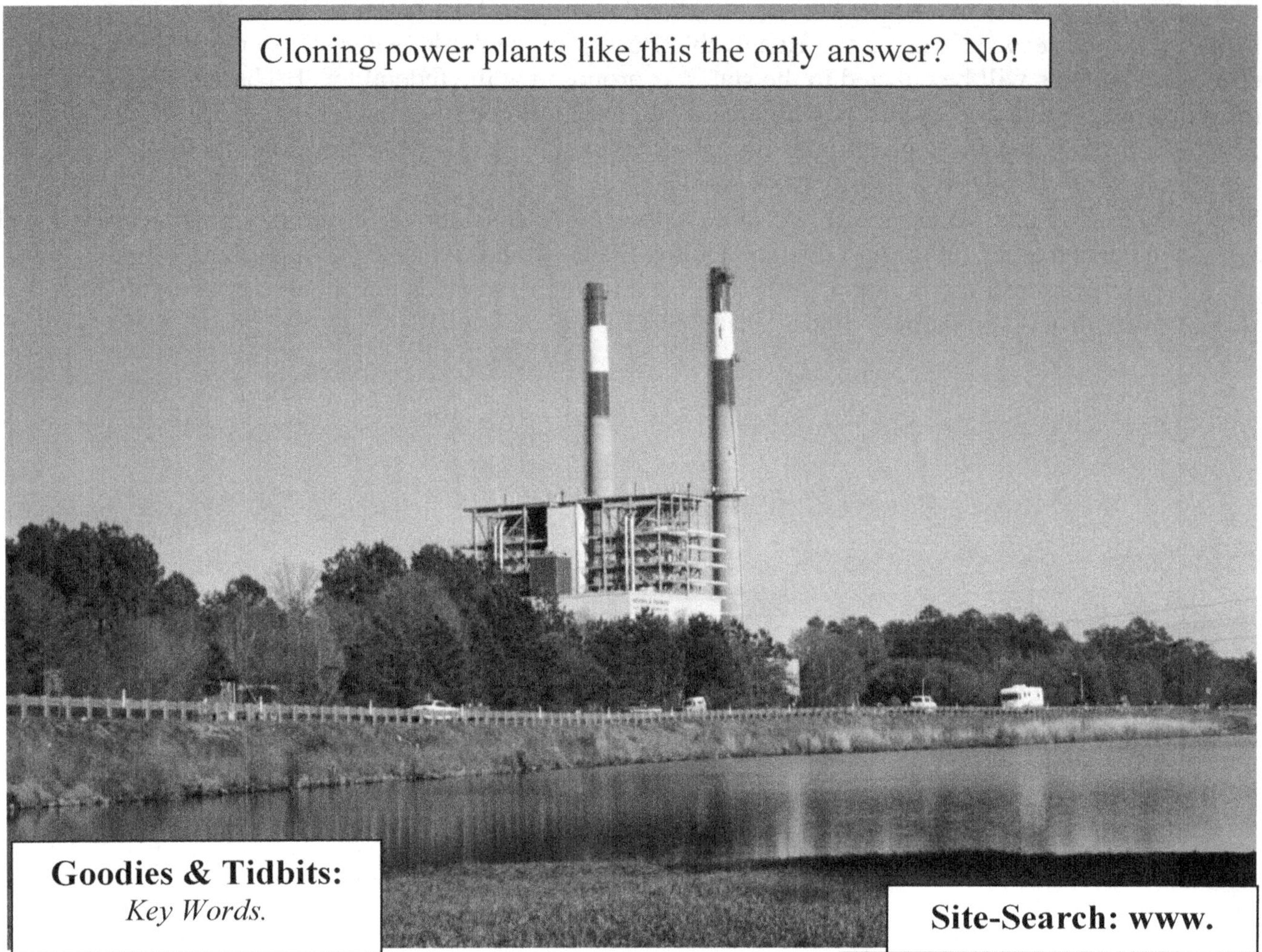

Goodies & Tidbits:

Key Words.

- **R**enewable **P**ortfolio **S**tandards
- Fuel Cells
- Photovoltaic
- Solar Thermal Power
- Hydrogen energy

Site-Search: www.

Usnews.com

green-energy.org/states.html

Albert, why do Americans need **R**enewable **P**ortfolio **S**tandards.

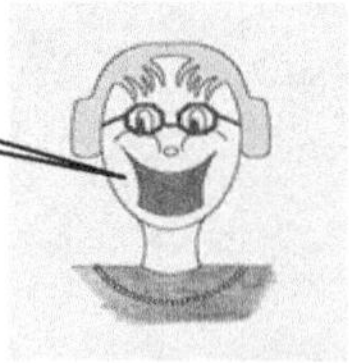

These "standards allow renewable forms of electrical generation to compete with the conventional methods. The cost of electrical production and environmental improvement are now going to be in the mix in determining the cost of electricity, which in the long run will create many public benefits, including environmental improvement, increased fuel diversity and national security, along with economic development." [23]

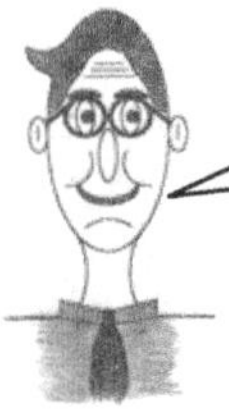

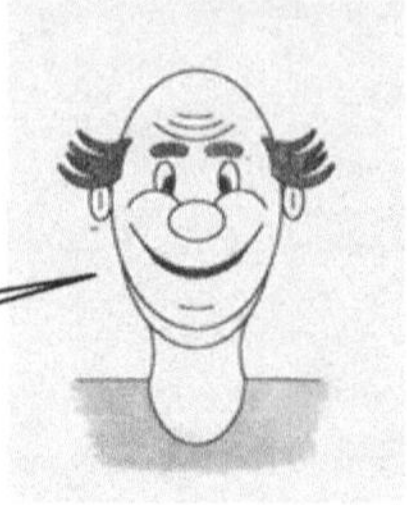

If they do what you're asking, Albert, there will be too much fresh air, and I don't trust any air I can't see.

Black Outs, Brown Outs!

New Ubiquitous Power Plants.

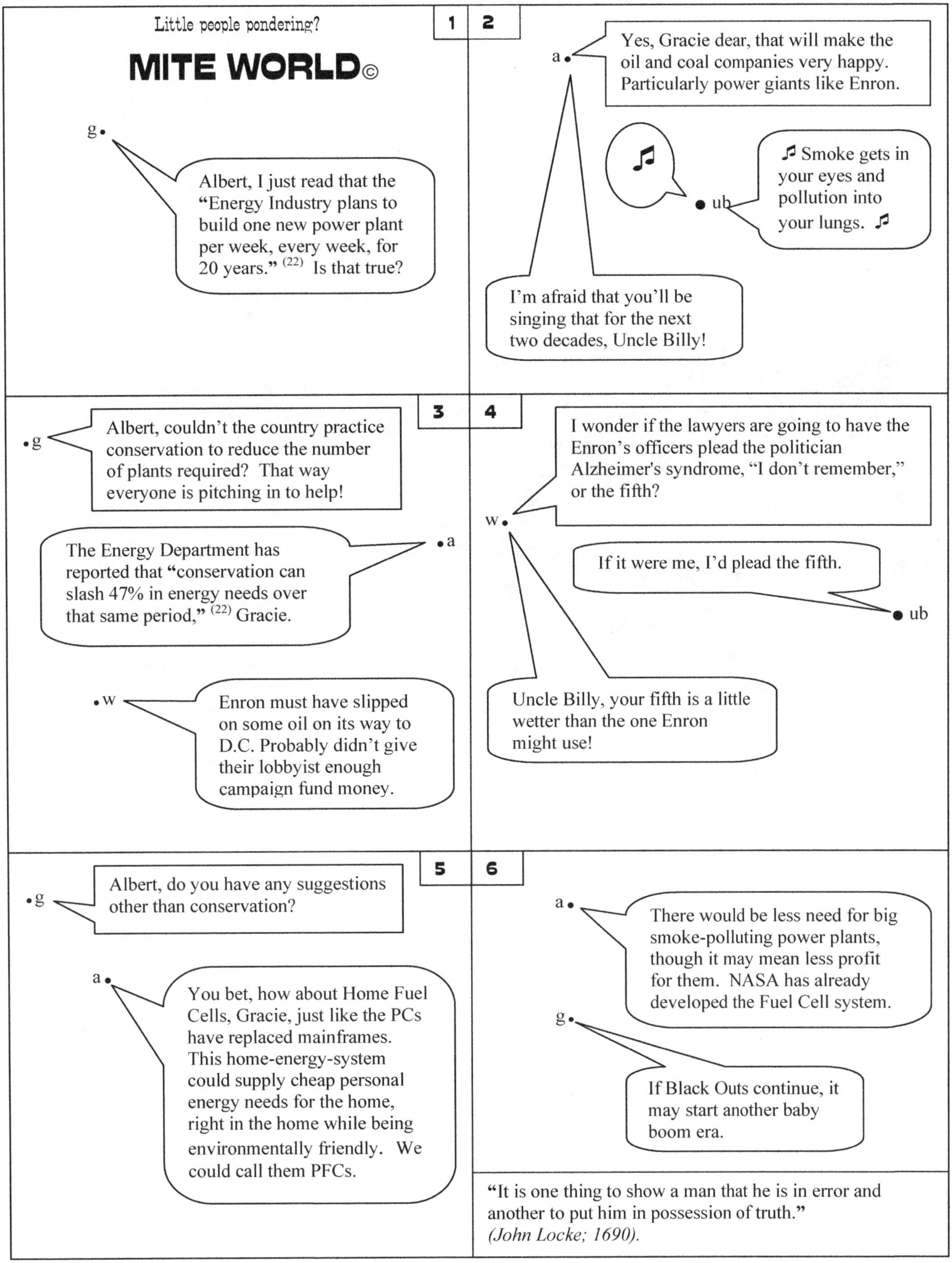

Goodbye Warbler- gone for ever

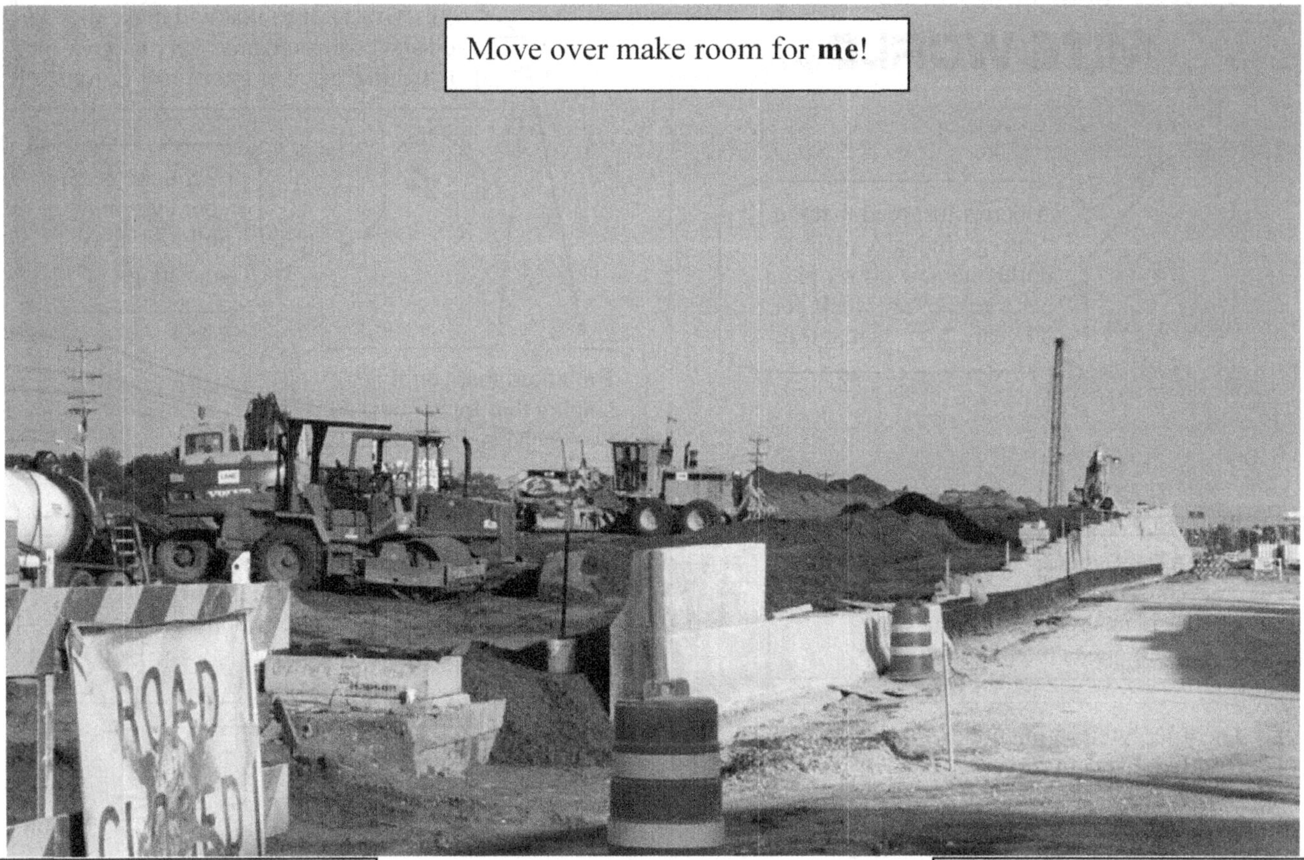

Goodies & Tidbits: *Key Words*
• Ecosystem • Keystone Species

Site-Search: www.
discover.com green-eergy.org/states.html

The World is losing 30,000 species/year!

Does anyone care?

Little people pondering?

MITE WORLD©

1

g: Albert, is it true that the ecological system is very delicate? The loss of one species can have a devastating ripple effect on all of us?

w: In the long past it was "cosmic accident or climate change causing much of the biological cataclysms. Now it is the marvelous narcissistic humans who alone are responsible for nearly every loss of species the past thousand years." (24)

2

a: Easy Walter! Yes Gracie dear, it is "estimated that for every one plant or animal that goes extinct, 15 other organisms will vanish." (24)

w: Albert, I have read it is "predicted that 50% of all living species could be lost in the next 50 years." (24)

a: Yes, Walter, hopefully Homo Sapiens aren't on that list!

3

w: I presume if man is not careful he might be on the return trip of Darwin's path of evolution!

g: Albert, what or who is destroying all this precious life?

a: Man is, Gracie. To meet the demands of the growing population, we are clearing land for housing and agriculture, replacing diverse wild plants with just a few varieties of crops, and introducing new chemicals into the environment.

4

a: This is occurring to the point where "experts estimate we're killing 30,000 species each year. Mostly insects— that thrive in tropical rain forests." (24)

ub: **Ugh!** Bugs again. Why worry about all that? Getting rid of bugs sounds like a good idea to me! I would enjoy my beer at the barbeque more if there were less of them.

a: Uncle Billy, "insects make the world as we know it work. They play a crucial role in pollination, they devour debris, and contain pests." (24)

ub: **Yeah! Yeah!** Bugs are OK I guess.

5

a: "To understand how ecological systems stay healthy, biologists study so-called keystone species, whose behavior helps shape the distinctive features of an ecosystem." (24)

g: Albert can you give some examples?

a: Yes, the "sea otter controls the population of sea urchins that feed on kelp, thus protecting kelp forests, which in turn shelter a variety of marine life and protect coastlines from wave erosion." (24)

6

a: Another interesting one is that "some seeds will not germinate unless they have passed through an elephant's digestive system first." (24)

ub: **Whoa!** Stop right there

w: I wager man doesn't know what species is a keystone until it's gone and takes others with it.

a: You got it!

Any man makes mistakes, but only an idiot persists in his errors. (Cicero; 43 BC.)

9.1.1

On September 11, 2001, America contacted a disease called terrorism brought here by Bin Laden and incorporated. To Prez Bush's credit he reacted quickly to eradicate the infestation. Though this is a short-term solution.

Destroying Bin Laden is only treating the symptom not the real disease. I wish there was an answer to counteracting hatred, prejudice and envy. Something is needed to sway the thinking of the world's masses while preventing more destruction. The eye for an eye only perpetuates hatred and killing. This has been done for centuries and doesn't work.

Maybe a pluralistic approach where in addition to fighting terrorists to keep them at bay, an all out humanitarian effort to help the world's health problems by the have nations for the have nots. Also a massive multifaceted message by all media's to project what is being done to help the world and denounce the terrorists who are disrupting the peace. This would be similar to the Voice-of-America, but could be changed to Voice-of-Earth. Much of the problem is the ignorance of the people supporting the likes of Bin Ladens. Maybe this is being naïve. Just a pondering?

The peaceful life before 911

Innocence destroyed

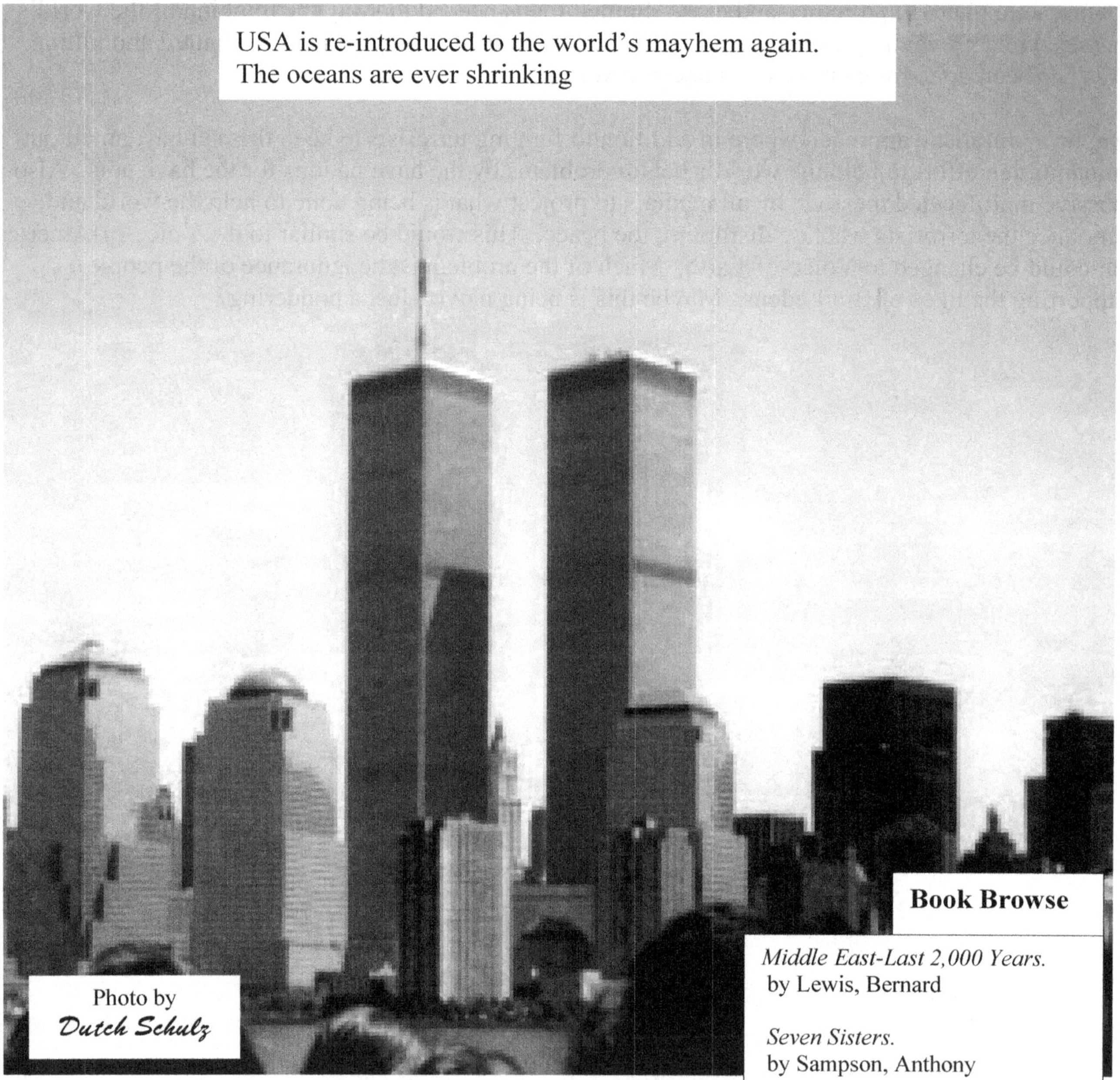

Photo by *Dutch Schulz*

Book Browse

Middle East-Last 2,000 Years.
by Lewis, Bernard

Seven Sisters.
by Sampson, Anthony

Crusades- The First Holy Wars,
US News, Arril 8, 2001

Part I, Bin Laden attacks America.

Hatred that begot Terror.

1

Little people pondering?

MITE WORLD©

ub: Is he the bad guy that wears a black hat?

g: No Uncle Billy, he wears a turban

g: Albert, why do he and his followers hate America so much?

2

a: There is no simple answer, Gracie, dear. The problems that we are living with at present are of course remnants of the past.

a: Well, Uncle Billy, let me give you a condensed version.

ub: Please explain? I'm confused, why anyone would kill himself to destroy a building with thousands of people in it.

3

a: Historically in the Muslim world there existed a "perpetual and obligatory state of war with its infidel neighbors." (25) These attitudes have lingered with the masses. In the Middle Ages they were a superior culture, but the Islamic nations grew complacent and stagnant while western Europe developed through industrialization and world exploration. The modernized European nations acquired global control of commerce and began to dominate the Middle East in the form of protectorates.

w: I'm sure that this didn't endear the West.

4

a: Being that their government and religion are integrated they resisted modernization or anything secular.

ub: **Wow!** Talk about a mouth full. Almost sorry I asked. That's condensed?

w: One of the best things our country's forefathers did was to separate religion and state.

ub: One good thing came out of the Twin Towers bombing is that more youngsters learned the words to the National Anthem.

5

a: To compete, the Muslim nations tried adapting Western ways, but religious leaders saw this as encroachment on their faith and "believing this the work of Satan." (25) This was implanted in the masses and has lasted for generations to the present time to explode with the radical Bin Laden against America.

ub: What a pest. Wish we could just use a bug spray to get rid of him!

g: It's hard to think that such animosity can live for so long.

6

a: Uncle Billy, Bin Laden is a religious fanatic who grew up in a region of the world that was exposed to imperialism by the West and was filled with hate. His hatred grew when America sent troops to Saudi Arabia during the Gulf War, believing that these troops from an alien culture were trespassing on his holy land. He used this as an excuse to appoint himself as a despotic leader to create a global Islamic state to fight the West. He has the money, resources and like Hitler the talent to misdirect people with lies to follow him in their mutual religious fervency and animosity of all things Western.

The Comeback after 911.

Affirmation of strength

Ground Zero: Dec 2001-a new generation proves its resolve.

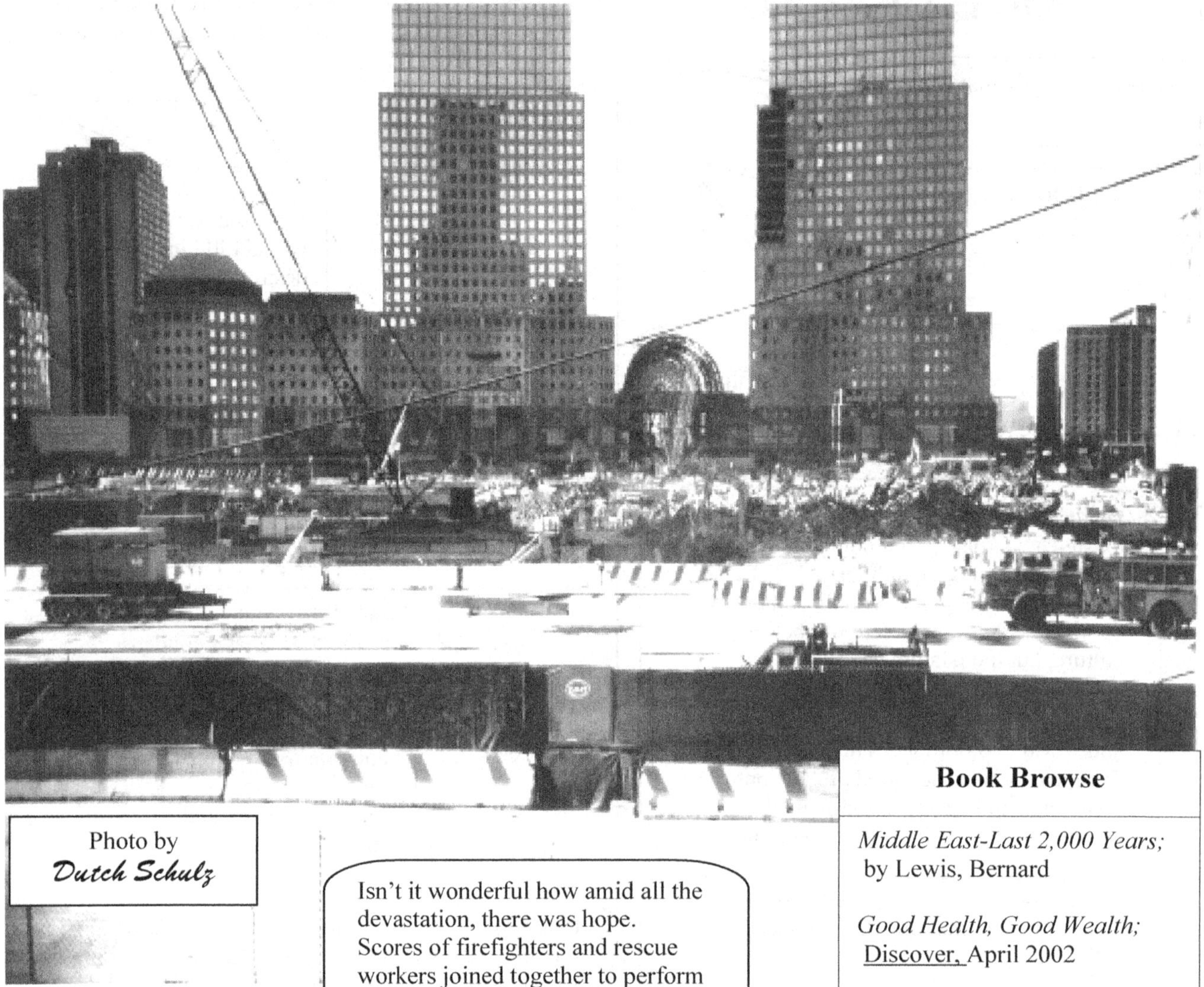

Photo by
Dutch Schulz

Book Browse

Middle East-Last 2,000 Years; by Lewis, Bernard

Good Health, Good Wealth; Discover, April 2002

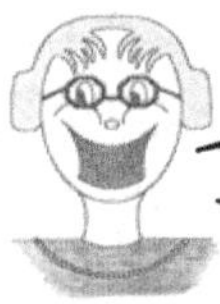

Isn't it wonderful how amid all the devastation, there was hope. Scores of firefighters and rescue workers joined together to perform a minor miracle of resurrection.

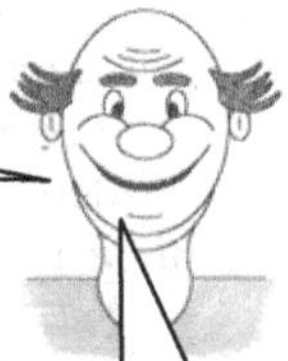

Boy, did the nation burst open with patriotism and flags waving all over in a show of strength and support.

Also,around the nation candle light memorial services were held to pray for the victims and show solidarity.

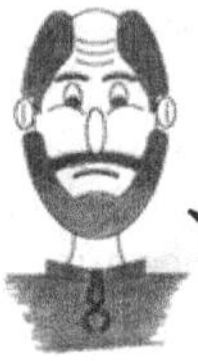

It's difficult for outsiders to understand how diversified independently minded Americans with all of our many disagreements and squabbles pull together in times of crisis.

Yeah! We Americans like being tidy. Clean up that mess and rebuild for a fresh start.

Part II, America attacks Bin Laden

Response to terrorist.

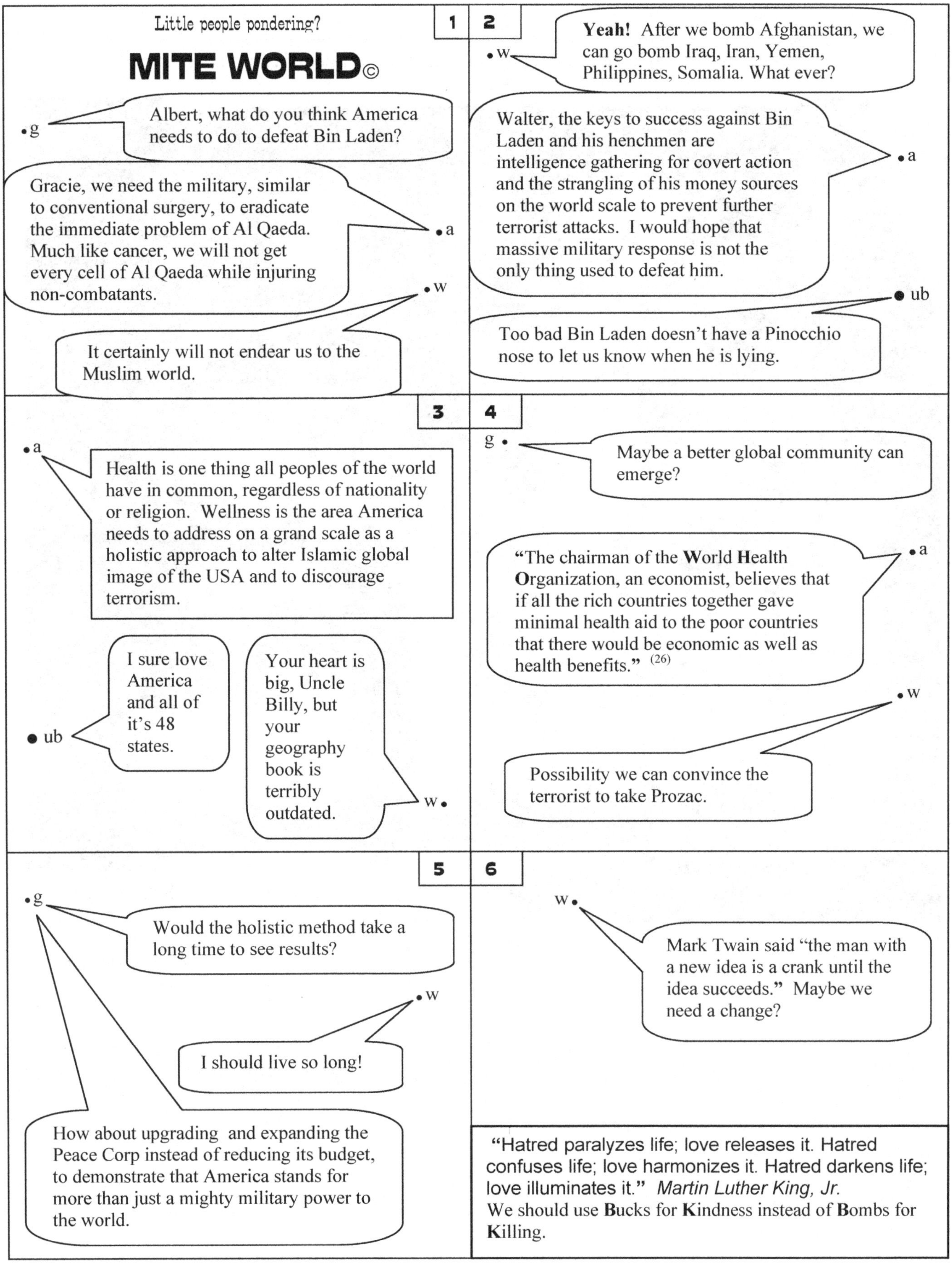

Chess is a pleasurable game, War is a horrific reality.

Chess & War both take patience, tactics and decisiveness.
But, Oh what a difference!

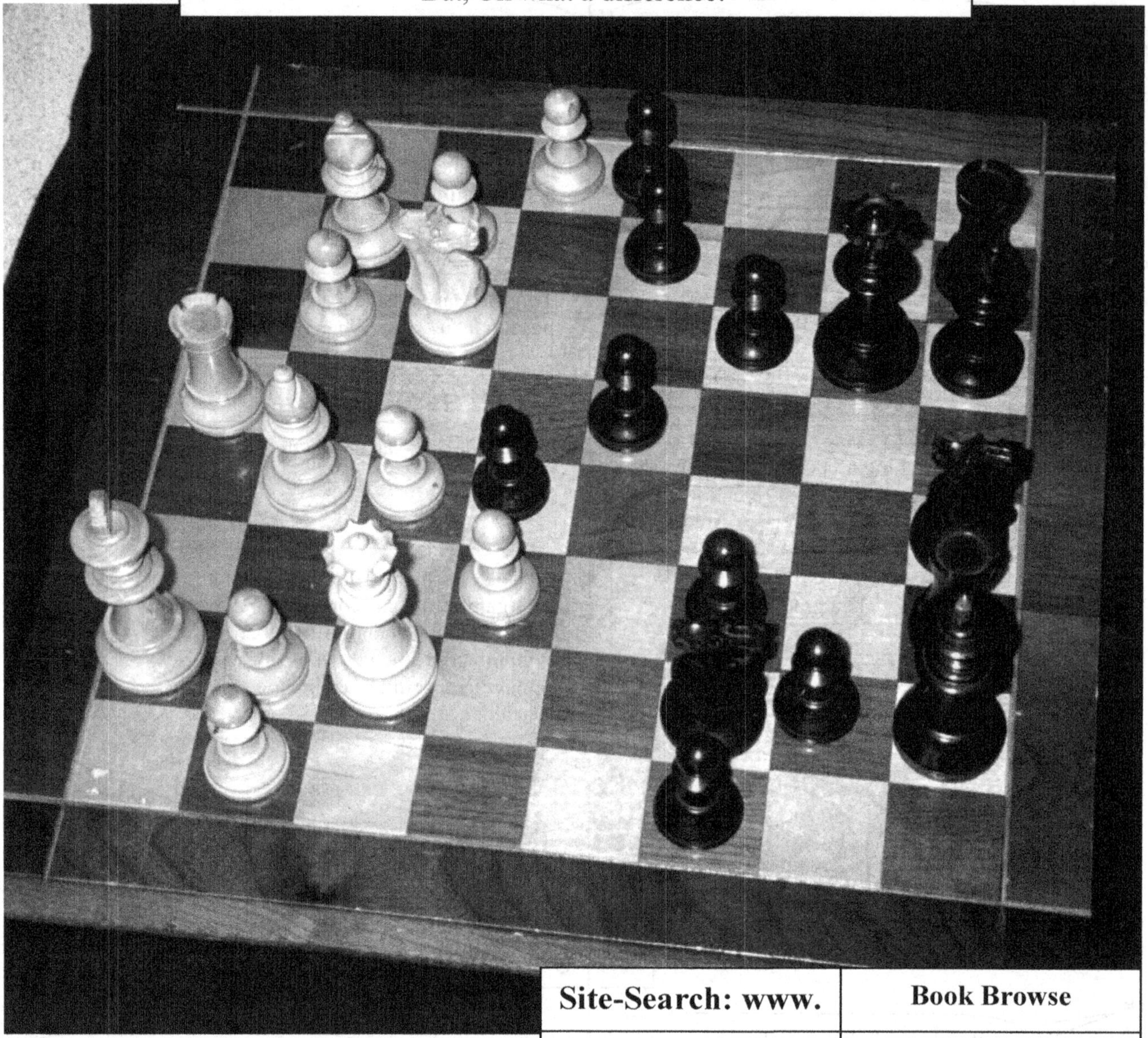

Site-Search: www.	Book Browse
discover.com	*Shield of Dreams;* Discover, November 2001 by Tim Folger

Antiballistic System

Shelter of dreams or is it nightmares?

1

Little people pondering?

MITE WORLD©

w: I heard that it is like trying to hit a bullet with another bullet.

This could be like the man who invented the boomerang. He got hurt on his first test. He forgot to duck.

g: Albert, does America really need an Antiballistic system?

2

a: Well Gracie dear, Prez Bush wants an Antiballistic system. Maybe this is his Texas upbringing of hooten and shooten macho image and leftover Cold War mentality. I don't think that it is a realistic idea.

w: We certainly don't need another Cuban crisis standoff!

ub: Sounds like the shoot out at the OK coral again.

3

a: I agree, Walter. You play chess and know that at times you move the pieces strategically to apply pressure about the board without ever intending to capture any pieces immediately. The problem with this is that your opponent sees this and may misinterpret thereby making an aggressive move you didn't want.

ub: Is this where an antiballistic system comes in?

4

a: Yes, Uncle Billy. Each side seeks to develop a shield to protect themselves against a missile attack with an antiballistic system.

Getting back to your question, Gracie, No! The difficulties with an antiballistic system are many, so much so that only a limited defense is now being planned mostly against single missile attacks and not MIRVs.

ub: What are MIRVs, some kind of disease like VD?

5

a: Well, Uncle Billy, much more dangerous, that stands for **M**ultiple **I**ndependently targetable **R**eentry **V**ehicles, a missile that can fire many warheads at a time before crashing into the earth.

w: It appears to be a form of white-collar welfare jobs.

g: Albert, are you against this system because it is so difficult to make it work?

6

a: Gracie, it's not only an unfeasible feat. It's not cost effective. The real danger is not ballistic missiles, since it would be cheaper and easier for an enemy to sail a boat loaded with an A-bomb into one of our harbors. How is an antiballistic missile going to help then? Particularly now with rampant Terrorists. "There are three phases at which to intercept a missile in flight, the boost, midcourse and reentry each with its own major problems. Worse yet is that the reaction time required is so rapid that only a computerized detection system will stand a chance of working, hence humans are out of the decision loop." [27]

"This is a hard and precarious world where every mistake and infirmity must be paid in full."
Clarence Day; 1920.

Bibliography

1.Goldberg, Burton. MD. Alternative Medicine the Definitive Guide. Tiburon, CA. Future Medicine Publishing, Inc.,1999, p.3-7 ***Convent vs. Holist***

2. Thimerosal – News. "Autism" Available http://www.thimerosal-news.com, May7, 2002 **Charts**

3. Mercola, Joseph MD. "Doctors are the 3rd leading cause of death." Available http://www.mercola.com, May22,2001 ***Charts***

4. Health Sciences Inst. Editorial Panel. "New breakthroughs against heart disease & stroke." Health Sciences Inst. report, Baltimore, Agora Publishing, Inc., 2001,p.1-4. **Cholesterol**

5. Whitaker, Julian MD. "Healthy alternatives to the 100 Most commonly prescribed drugs." Health & Healing report, Potomac, MD. Phillips Publishing, Inc., 1999 pg.53-54. **Cholesterol**

6. Douglass, W.C. MD. "Slash your risk of Alzheimer's overnight." Available. http://www.whale.to/d/fluoride3.html. 2002. ***Alzheimer's***

7. Null, Gary, PhD. "Introduction to the fluoridation issue." Available http:// www.garynull.com. 2002. ***Alzheimer's***

8. Surgeon General. "Report on consequences of smoking." Available http:// www.cdc.gov\tobacco. 1964. ***Butts***

9. Goldberg, Burton MD. Alternative Medicine the Definitive Guide. Tiburon, CA. Future Medicine Publishing, Inc. 1999, pg. 20-21, 566-575 **Cancer Crime**

10. Health Sciences Inst. Editorial Panel. "How you can take advantage of the AMAS cancer test." Available http://www.agora-inc.com Feb22, 2002. **Cancer Test**

11. Oncolab, Inc. "AMAS cancer test." Available http://www.amascancertest.com, Feb22, 2002. **Cancer Test**

12. Health Sciences Inst. Editorial Panel. "Stronger than steroids: new solutions for beating arthritis." Health Sciences Inst. report, Baltimore, Agora Publishing, Inc, 2001,p.1-7 **Arthritis Part I & II**

13. Whitaker, Julian MD. "Healthy alternatives to the 100 Most commonly prescribed drugs." Health & Healing report, Potomac, MD. Phillips Publishing, Inc., 1999,p.43-45 **Arthritis Part I & II**

14. Batmanhelidj, F. MD. Your body's many cries for water. Falls Church, VA. Global Health Solutions Inc.,1997,p.8-11 **Dehydration.**

15. Johnson, R Jill. Oxycise. Conifer, CO. Oxycise International, Inc., Distributed by Guthy-Renker, 1997, pg.1-86 **Oxygen.**

16. Williams, David PhD. "Volume8 #23". Alternatives Newsletter. Potomac, MD. Mountain Home Publishing, May 2001 pg.177-179. **Advertising**

17.Barry, Patricia. "Ads, promotions drive up costs". AARP Bulletin, March 2002. p.1,3 Washington DC **Advertising**

18. Douglass, W.C. MD. Into the Light. Atlanta. Second Opinion Publishing Inc, 1993,p.291-293 ***Sunlight***

19. Goldberg, Burton MD. Alternative Medicine the Definitive Guide. Tiburon, CA. Future Medicine Publishing, Inc.,1999,p. 168-170. **Additives**

20. Greenberg, Gary. "The Sertorin surprise." Discover, July 2001, p.84-89. **T*een Violence***

21. Whitaker, Julian MD. "Antidepressants." Health & Healing report, Potomac, MD. Phillips Publishing, Inc., 2001. **TeenViolence.**

Bibliography

22. Whitman, David. "Power up the power plants." US News & World Report, May 21, 2001. ***Blackouts***

23. Union of concerned scientist. "Renewable portfolio standard" Available http://www.green-energy/states.html, May11,2002. ***Blackouts***

24. McClintock, Jack. "Twenty Species We May Lose in the Next 20 Years." Discover, Oct. 2000. ***Species***

25. Bernard, Lewis. The Middle East-Last 2,000 Years. New York NY. Touchstone, 1995 **Terror Parts I &II**

26. Sachs, Jeffrey. "Good Health, Good Wealth." Discover, Apr. 2002, p.16 ***Terror Part II***

27. Folger, Tim. "Shield of Dreams" Discover, Nov. 2001, **Antiballistic**

28. G. Perret with T. Martin. Little Giant Encyclopedia of One Liners. New York. Sterling Publishing Co. Inc., 1999

Little people a pondering?

Mite World © 2002

Visit Mite World on the web & Continue to Chuckle your way down the Path to Wellness

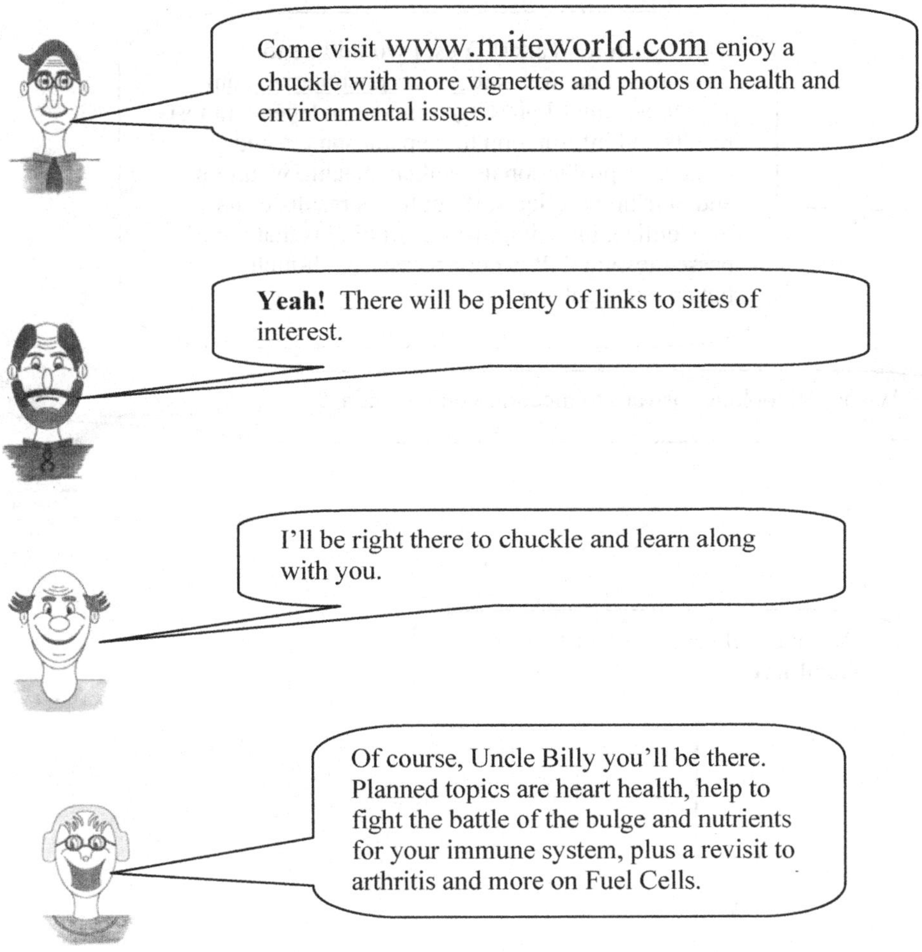

Finale.

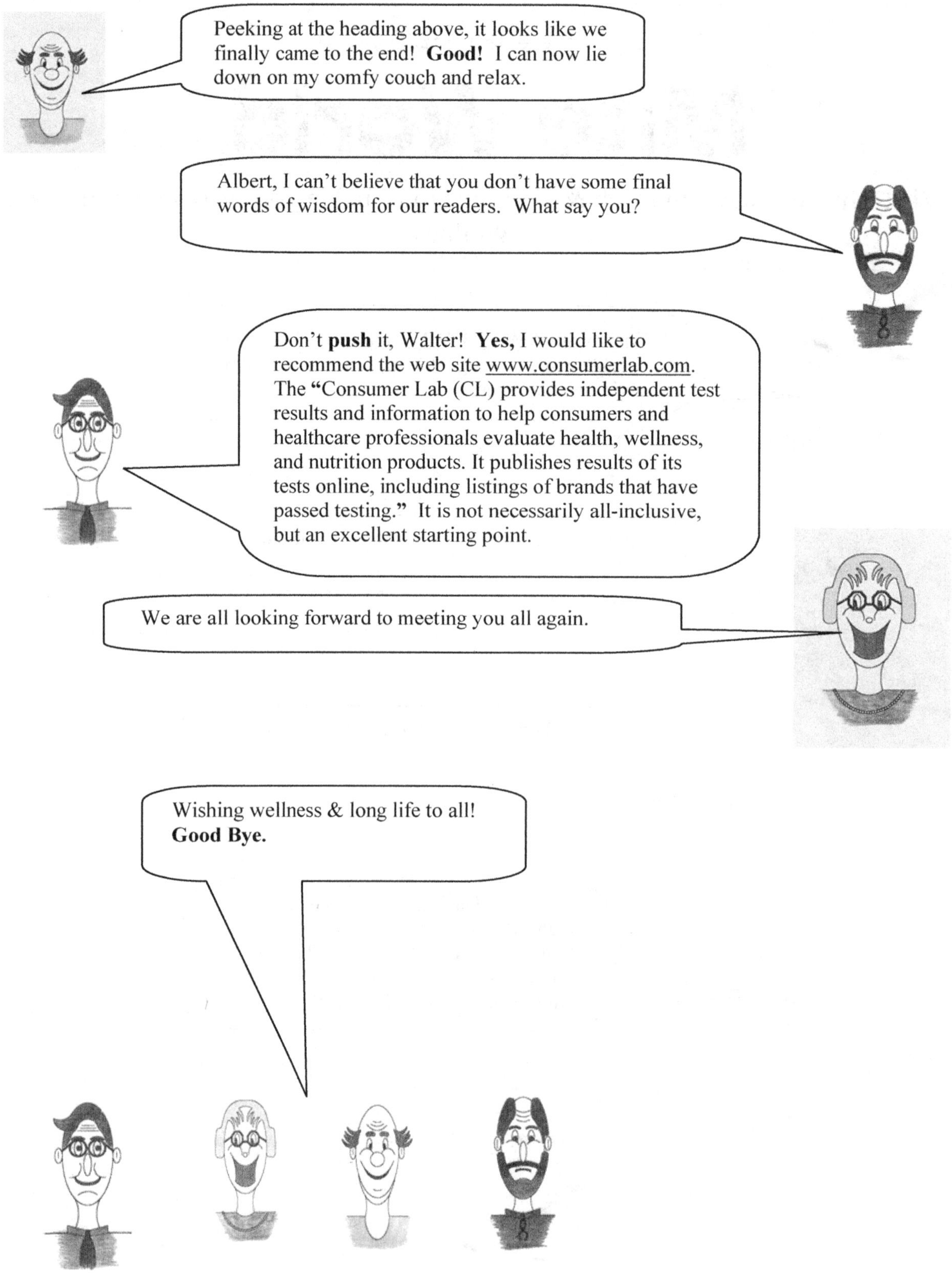
Peeking at the heading above, it looks like we finally came to the end! **Good!** I can now lie down on my comfy couch and relax.
Albert, I can't believe that you don't have some final words of wisdom for our readers. What say you?
Don't **push** it, Walter! **Yes,** I would like to recommend the web site www.consumerlab.com. The "Consumer Lab (CL) provides independent test results and information to help consumers and healthcare professionals evaluate health, wellness, and nutrition products. It publishes results of its tests online, including listings of brands that have passed testing." It is not necessarily all-inclusive, but an excellent starting point.
We are all looking forward to meeting you all again.
Wishing wellness & long life to all! **Good Bye.**

Made in the USA
Monee, IL
08 November 2026

67378660R00037